For Bill Bates MD

I wanted to share this book which 2 classmates and I wrote to commemorate and memorialize a great mentor with a dear friend, and also a mentor to me.

Bill Corley

Ray E. Brown
Lectures, Messages, and Memoirs

Ray E. Brown
Lectures, Messages, and Memoirs

EDITED BY
Mary M. Blanks
William E. Corley
S. Douglas Smith

Foreword by J. Alexander McMahon

Health Administration Press
Ann Arbor, Michigan

95 94 93 92 91 5 4 3 2 1

Library of Congress Cataloging-in-Publication Data

Ray E. Brown : lectures, messages, and memoirs / edited by Mary M. Blanks, William E. Corley, S. Douglas Smith; preface by J. Alexander McMahon.
p. cm.
Includes bibliographical references.
ISBN 0-910701-68-7 (alk. paper)
1. Brown Ray E. 2. Hospital administrators—United States—Biography. I. Brown, Ray E. II. Blanks, Mary M. III. Corley, William E. IV. Smith, S. Douglas.
[DNLM: 1. Brown, Ray E. 2. Hospital Administration—biography. WZ 100 B8794]
RA971.B85R39 1991 362.1'1'068—dc20 [B]
DNLM/DLC for Library of Congress 90-15656 CIP

Health Administration Press
A division of the Foundation of the
American College of Healthcare Executives
1021 East Huron Street
Ann Arbor, Michigan 48104-9990
(313) 764-1380

We dedicate this book in memory of
RAY E. BROWN

There is no doubt that he has changed the lives of each of us who knew and studied under him. By the pages of this volume we, his students, hope that those who follow us, not having the privilege of being able to attend his classes, will nevertheless be able to acquaint themselves with the traditions for which he stood and profit as we have from his example.

Contents

Preface

This book is a result of love and admiration: love for a great teacher by former students at Duke; admiration for a faculty colleague, co-worker, and contemporary by a number of people who encouraged the former students in their efforts and added their own tribute to one of the giants of the field of hospital administration.

Ray Everett Brown was indeed, as David Kinzer describes him in Part Two, a "triple threat," combining "preeminence in teaching," "big league experience in institutional management," and "top level political leadership in his field."

Ray was a great teacher, not only in the classrooms at Chicago and Duke, but also through his writings. His former students, Mary Blanks, Bill Corley, and Doug Smith, have performed a great service by recording for administrative posterity two of Ray's "three interwoven processes" of the practice of administration. He had recorded one in his book, *Judgment in Administration*, published in 1966; the other two, "turn of mind" and "administrative strategies," form the core of Part One of this book. Mary, Bill, and Doug explain the development of these three chapters in the Introduction to Part One.

Part Two describes his experiences in management and political leadership, seen through the eyes of some of his many admirers and close professional associates. With one exception, all of the contents of Part Two were written by request, as part of the design of a new book. The one exception is "Ray E. Brown: Prototype Hospital Administrator," written by Aaron Cohodes in 1962 when Ray had just arrived at one of his career peaks. It is still counted among the best articles about Ray ever written.

Ray was an excellent administrator, with varied experience at Chicago, Duke, Harvard, and Northwestern. His approaches to administration at the University of Chicago are chronicled in Chapters Four and Five. The Duke years, and the development of the master's degree program in hospital administration there, are covered in Chapter Six. The Harvard and Northwestern experiences are described in Chapters Seven and Eight.

Ray's political leadership is apparent in the positions to which his peers elected him. He served as the chief elected officer of both the American Hospital Association and the American College of Hospital Administrators (now the American College of Healthcare Executives). There are now awards by both organizations given in his name. His American Hospital Association activities are described in Chapter Nine, and other evidence of his leadership is found in Chapter Ten, as told by a collection of people who worked with him over the years.

My own friendship with Ray began with his arrival at Duke in 1964. I was then Secretary-Treasurer of the North Carolina Association of County Commissioners, and since his first job was that of County Manager of Cleveland County, we had an immediate kinship. The counties of North Carolina had a substantial involvement in hospitals, so I was an invitee to the early Duke Forums which Ray began. The invitations, and the relationship, continued when I moved to Blue Cross and Blue Shield in North Carolina the following year. We met regularly during his Boston years, because he returned annually to the Duke Forums, and we became neighbors when I moved to Chicago and the American Hospital Association in late 1972.

Over the next year and a half, we visited occasionally, shared a couple of platforms, and traveled together once or twice. Our North Carolina background provided a bond, but it was strengthened by Ray's willingness to accept yet another student for his teaching of administration and political leadership. He approached administration as more art than science, an approach I found compatible with my own. Hence I encouraged the development of this book in its present form, particularly his former students' contribution in Part One. Yet, in my thinking, Part One needs the real life applications portrayed in Part Two, where one will find the teachings in action in administration and political leadership.

I think of Ray often. His picture graces the lobby of our health administration program offices and one of our students is aided by a scholarship named for him. To some readers, those who knew him, I hope this book is a reminder of a giant in the field. To others who had not the privilege of knowing him, I hope it offers the lessons that his students and friends learned firsthand.

A word about the contributors. "Part One, Ray E. Brown: the Teacher," was compiled by three graduates of the Duke Program in Hospital Administration, students of Ray Brown in the 1960s. Mary M. Blanks until recently was Assistant Commissioner of the Department of Mental Health, State of Oklahoma, in Oklahoma City; William E. Corley is President, Community Hospitals of Indiana, Inc., Indianapolis, Indiana; and S. Douglas Smith is President, Quorum Health Resources, Inc., Nashville, Tennessee.

In addition to Aaron Cohodes, contributors to Part Two are Richard L. Johnson, President of Tribrook, Inc., Hospital Consultants, of Oak Brook, Illinois; Donald S. Smith, Assistant Professor of Health Administration, Duke University; Richard Wittrup, for many years a member of the consulting firm of Herman Smith and Associates, now working at the Henry Ford Hospital in Detroit; Robert Cunningham, former editor of *Modern Hospital* magazine and now an editorial consultant for the Blue Cross and Blue Shield Association, Chicago; George Bugbee, for many years the Chief Executive of the American Hospital Association and, later, professor and head of the graduate program in hospital administration at the University of Chicago; James E. Hague, for many years editor of *Hospitals*, the journal of the American Hospital Association; and the late David Kinzer, former president of the Massachusetts Hospital Association, who was a lecturer in the School of Public Health, Harvard University, and in the Department of Health Administration, Duke University.

Finally, a strong word of appreciation to Bob Cunningham and David Kinzer, both of whom helped edit the final product and brought it into publishable form.

J. Alexander McMahon
Durham, North Carolina
May 1989

Biographical Note

Ray Everett Brown
1913–1974

Ray Everett Brown was born in Union, South Carolina, on September 26, 1913, the son of the Reverend William Thomas and Fan Casey Brown. Rev. Brown was a Baptist minister who moved with his family from one community to another several times during Ray Brown's early years, while Ray attended country schools in the Carolinas. When he finished high school Ray enrolled at Gardner Webb College, a Southern Baptist preparatory school at Boiling Springs, North Carolina, and after two years there enrolled at the University of North Carolina at Chapel Hill, where he graduated in 1937 with a B.S. degree in accounting. This knowledge of accounting got him his first job as county manager of Cleveland County, North Carolina, and led to his appointment as superintendent of the Shelby, North Carolina, Hospital in 1940. At Shelby, Ray was comfortable managing hospital finances but aware that he lacked anything more than a superficial understanding of other phases of hospital operation. That lack of understanding prompted him to sign up for an institute or "short course" in hospital management at the University of Chicago. At the institute, Ray's searching questions drew the attention of Dr. Arthur C. Bachmeyer, superintendent of university hospitals and director of the graduate program in hospital administration, and a nationally recognized leader of the emerging profession.

They talked at length, and Dr. Bachmeyer told Ray that what he needed for a successful career in hospital administration was the thorough, all-around knowledge and understanding afforded by graduate study.

Ray was convinced. He returned to Shelby, loaded his family and their possessions into the car and drove to Chicago, where he finished a year's study and the required practicum in something less than the usual two years. He went back to North Carolina with an M.B.A. in hospital administration, and a job as superintendent of North Carolina Baptist Hospital at Winston-Salem.

In 1945 Dr. Bachmeyer invited Ray to come back as superintendent of the university's hospitals and clinics. He spent the next nineteen years at the University of Chicago as administrator of the university's general and special teaching hospitals, as assistant professor and then professor of hospital administration, assistant director and then director of the graduate program in hospital administration in the university's school of business and, as vice-president of the university, in charge of all its business operations. He didn't particularly enjoy the last assignment: it took him away from the hospital/medical environment that had been his life's interest for so many years, and that made every day an adventure to be relished. In addition, the university was growing, and a large part of Ray's time in the new job as vice-president had to be spent negotiating for city property adjacent to the campus and dealing with contractors, as well as university departments, on details of building plans and costs.

When an opportunity came to get back to where he felt he belonged, Ray moved on to become a professor of administration and director of the graduate program in hospital administration at Duke University. Ray Brown might readily and happily have stayed at Duke until he retired. But an old friend whose appeal for help he could not refuse decided matters differently. This friend was Robert Ebert, M.D., who had been an assistant professor of medicine at the University of Chicago when Ray came to the hospitals. An extraordinary young man who had taken a degree in philosophy after he finished medical school, Dr. Ebert became professor of medicine and head of the department. He and Ray saw each other regularly for ten years and they became good friends, their talks starting and ending with hospitals but roaming the expanse of human behavior. Ebert went on to Western Reserve and University Hospitals in Cleveland, and then to Harvard, where he was professor of medicine, dean of the medical school, and head of the department of medicine at Massachusetts General Hospital. In 1967, when he called Ray Brown at Duke, the merger of teaching hospitals and the planning of the new affiliated hospitals to replace the old Peter Bent Brigham Hospital had been seen as needed but remained to be accomplished. Plainly, Harvard needed a firm hand at the hospital helm, and Ebert was sure he knew where to get one. "You'll have to come," he told Ray, and Ray came.

Some years later, he told a friend, "The best way to accomplish a hospital merger would be to get the needed signatures on the documents that are legally required, and not tell anybody else until it was done." The more people who know about it in advance, the more trouble you'll have getting it done, he said, because they all think they may have something to lose. At Harvard, in addition to the internal complexities, the neighborhood was up in arms. The plan for the new affiliated hospitals building meant that a row of old residences, many of them made over into rooming houses, had to come down, and public turmoil had resulted. This was in the late 1960s when the civil rights movement was at its apex, with leaders who knew how to make the most of a struggle that could be presented as "the establishment" against "the people." The tensions were formidable. "There were days when Ray had to cross picket lines to get to his office," an assistant related.

The picket lines on Boston streets didn't trouble Ray Brown as much as the picket lines inside the heads of those who feared loss of identity in the contemplated merger. As he had in Chicago as vice-president for administration, Ray was spending too much of his time, as he saw it, resolving difficulties that had little to do with the consuming interest of his career, and when the right kind of occasion was presented, he responded and moved on. As executive vice president of the McGaw Medical Center at Northwestern University in Chicago he was among old friends, creating the organization to make an efficient operating entity of the five hospitals that were its principal components.

Engaged as he had been with his responsibilities at the University of Chicago and at Duke, Harvard, and Northwestern, Ray Brown always had time to write the papers he presented at meetings of state, regional, and national associations of hospital administrators, and to be an active participant in association affairs. Accountants are not invariably noted for the precision and clarity of their prose, but Ray was a notable exception; his contributions to the literature of his profession were widely sought after and acclaimed. His active membership and participation in professional organizations is evident from his selection as president and board member of both the American Hospital Association (AHA) and the American College of Hospital Administrators. Moreover, both organizations honored him for outstanding professional contributions, the AHA with its Distinguished Service Award in 1963 and the College with the Gold Medal Award in 1969.

Ray Brown's counsel was valued in a wide range of professional and related activities. Thus he was a consultant to the Surgeon General of the Army and the Surgeon General of the Air Force, a member of the executive committee of the White House Conference on Health in 1965 and the national advisory committee of the National Conference on the Costs of Medical Care convened by President Lyndon Johnson in 1967; he was member of the Joint Commission on the Accreditation of Hospitals, the National Commission on Nursing and Nursing Education, the National Commission to Study Medical Education, and the National Task Force on Health Facilities. He was also active in community affairs beyond the boundaries of his interest in health, as a member of the Board of Directors of the Blue Cross Plan of Chicago, a member of the board and president of the University of Chicago Settlement, a trustee of the Home for Destitute Crippled Children, a director of the Chicago Welfare Council, a member of the executive committee of the Chicago Community Fund, and a director of the National Council on Philanthropy. Ray was a member of the board of directors of the American Sterilizer Corporation and Parke-Davis and Company. He was an interested observer of business operations. As a friend who owned his own business remarked, "Ray's ideas were brilliant, and his advice was always sound; his impatience with the difficulties we encountered gaining acceptance of new ideas and selling products was consistent with the character that would have made him an outstanding success as a businessman."

Ray Brown suffered a coronary occlusion and died in May 1974. He is still missed as the leading figure of his profession in his time, but his work goes on in the accomplishments of the hundreds who were his students and associates over the years.

Part One

Ray E. Brown: The Teacher

INTRODUCTION

In 1976 we three former students of Ray Brown began the time-consuming task of putting into publishable form his unpublished notes and papers. Our purpose was to share his unique ideas and perceptions on management with practicing managers and students who did not have the good fortune to know him either as a student or a peer. We wanted to preserve, for ourselves and others, the ideas he had intended to publish at the time of his death. As we began to review his papers we saw, based on the handwriting and in some cases the sketchy notes, that our task was not going to be an easy one.

We analyzed his and our own notes on the two components of his theory on administration or management, the "turn of mind" or "administrative senses" of a good administrator, and the management strategies which all managers use, often without thinking about using a specific strategy.

Those who knew Ray Brown personally and know his precise writing style will appreciate the problem we had translating his notes and thoughts into meaningful sentences and paragraphs that he would agree conveyed his true meaning. The first portions of the two following chapters were actually written by him. It is probably obvious that the second portions were our attempts to reconstruct the chapters from our notes.

This process of reconstruction has consumed more than ten years. The three of us have become better friends and colleagues through this process. The sharing of ideas, the constant questioning of "did he really mean this?" took a lot of time. We hope we have made this book a contribution close to what he would have made had he lived to finish his writing. We believe, fifteen years after Ray's death, that most of this material is just as relevant and useful to health management careerists as it was when we were his students.

"If all members of an enterprise could be expected to do spontaneously and automatically what is best for the organization," Brown has said, "there would not be justification to have administrative people. But such perfect group interaction simply does not exist. Therefore, I propose this theory: that administration has as its purpose the responsibility of causing behavior.

"To cause behavior is often an act of interfering with the good intentions of many people; this is done to secure appropriate, composite behavior that will yield the best results for the purpose of the organization."

Ray Brown believed the practice of management, or administration, involved three interwoven processes which, combined, enabled the manager to cause, contrive, or synthesize behavior. These three processes are (1) judgment, the subject of Brown's book, *Judgment in Administration*, published in 1966; (2) turn of mind, or the manner of thinking of the administrator, or, said another way, how the administrator thinks uniquely; and (3) strategy, the way the administrator implements a decision to achieve desired results. Two of these processes, turn of mind and strategy, are the subject of Part One of this book.

When Ray Brown described the art and craft of administration, he called it a "thinking man's game,"* "chauffeuring the apparatus," and "an intellectual process."

Brown believed that the administrator was not bound by personality, but rather must develop a second or administrative personality. A purpose of professional education is to enable the individual to develop this second personality, and failure to do so means the individual will not be fully able to see things according to the demands of the profession. The administrator must

---

*The use of "man" and the masculine pronouns throughout is more a sign of those times than of Brown's attitude.

develop a way of acting that is beyond the self, that is unique to an administrator.

Turn of mind is part of the second personality Brown referred to. It is the administrator's sense of administration, a blend of thinking. The administrator must be able to play an administrative role. Brown described 31 senses that make up the turn of mind of an effective administrator. Understanding and recognizing these senses give insight into how the administrator or manager thinks, and why he is unique. These senses are described in this book as Brown described them in his notes and lectures. The manager or reader will recognize many of his own characteristics and those he sees in other managers.

The administrator has a unique inventory of traits, and his ability to mix and use them enables him to take the "proper action at the proper time." The good administrator acts as he *should,* not always as he wishes.

The only tool an administrator has is what he knows and thinks. His unique turn of mind enables him to know that "two and two equals four without knowing the second two." It is the ability to know intuitively the difference between "prevailing winds and intermittent breezes." Brown often said, "If administration ever develops a coat of arms, it will be a question mark."

Turn of mind can be described as what the administrator sees and permits himself to see, what he feels and permits himself to feel. It is the total of all his attitudes that influences how his mind works; it is how he sees the world; and it sets the framework for how he understands and uses strategy.

The strategy chosen determines how a decision is implemented, and it is at this point that managers often fail. Brown believed that although a good decision was desirable, it was not absolutely necessary, since skillful use of strategy would enable the administrator to get a good result with even a poor decision.

Brown believed that human behavior must be changed or interfered with in order for the manager to get his way and, further, that the manager will be more successful in changing behavior if he can choose and use strategy skillfully. Strategy is how the administrator gets things done; it is "putting notions into effect." It is how the administrator gets results. Brown pointed out that the results obtained needed only to be adequate to satisfy the situation. That is, the *best* solution is not necessary, only a solution which will take care of the problem at hand. Recognizing what and how much is required and effectively carrying out appropriate actions are effective utilization of strategy.

In his papers and lectures, Brown described 42 strategies that will enable the administrator to produce desired results. Some strategies conflict with others; these strategies are a "shopping list" from which the administrator can pick and choose different strategies for different situations.

As the manager studies the strategies identified by Brown, he will begin to realize the ways and times when they can be utilized. Many, if not most, will be learned by the manager over the course of a long career. However, the manager who becomes a student of strategy early in his career has the benefit of this knowledge throughout the years.

Judgment is the third of the processes that Brown described, and the only one which resulted in a book. In *Judgment in Administration,* Brown states that "Good judgment is said to be the child of wisdom. This must mean that bad judgment has other parents." The book concerns those other parents because Brown believed that although the administrator usually has good judgment, it is his occasional bad judgment that is noticed. Brown also believed that although the administrator usually *has* good judgment, he doesn't always exhibit good judgment—and he is judged on the judgment he *exhibits.*

> Good judgment occurs when you have the ability to see the facts through the values of the people around you; that, of course, is what we call common sense. Common sense is the sense that people think they would have demonstrated if they had the same facts you had. To try to see the facts through the eyes of the other person does not mean that you abandon your own convictions, but it does give some insight into how to avoid mistakes . . . poor judgment results largely from an interference with the judgment process, and the exercise of good judgment depends in large part upon controlling the . . . interferences.
>
> The value of this book, *Judgment in Administration,* is in helping the reader to become more aware of these interferences with his judgment and to exert a conscious effort to

> control them. Watching them and controlling them is the administrator's best answer, for it is the only answer. He will never completely eliminate them.

Ray Brown meant to write a book on each of the three processes—turn of mind, strategy, and judgment—but only the judgment book was completed. This book has been written to give practicing administrators the opportunity to study and use Brown's ideas on the other two processes.

Without relentless pushing, encouragement, cajoling and emotional support from classmates and members of the Duke University faculty, the ideas contained in Brown's notes could not have evolved into publication form.

We also appreciate the help given us by the secretarial staff of the Hospital Corporation of America. We also would like to thank Mary Brown for permitting us to proceed with this publication. A portion of the proceeds from the book's sale will go to the Ray Brown Scholarship Fund at Duke University.

Mary M. Blanks
William E. Corley
S. Douglas Smith

Chapter One

The Turn of Mind of the Effective Administrator

The good administrator must have a good mind, but a good mind is not enough. It is the way the mind works that makes a good administrator. What one thinks about and the way one thinks about it are as important as the ability to think. There are different ways of thinking, and the administrator must think like a good administrator should if he is to be a good administrator.

Every profession has its own particular way of thinking. This is because it has its own particular responsibilities for which to do its thinking. Each professional has a manner of thinking that comes to prevail after a certain amount of thinking and experience in his particular profession. His thinking is bent to best serve his professional function. We talk of the legal mind, the medical mind, the banker's mind—and these do exist. The precise accountant's mind works differently from that of the sympathetic social worker, and the cautious banker's manner of thinking differs from that of the risk-taking entrepreneur. The science-oriented physician has a different mind-set from that of the faith-oriented minister. These differences in thinking are as they should be. They are necessary if the professional is to carry out his function effectively. The purpose of a profession is to provide differentiated thinking.

The mind is the major instrument of the professional, and he must use it according to the purposes of his profession. When he thinks professionally he is supposed to think purposefully. To do this he must develop a disposition to think about those things important to his function and to think about them in a way that is meaningful to it. This disposition must become so deeply imbedded in him that it becomes a "turn of mind." If his mind is not turned in keeping with the requirements of his professional purpose, he cannot expect to think about the most meaningful things in the most meaningful way. A person cannot change his way of thinking as one changes his shirt. Whether it fits his professional needs or not, every individual does have and does use a turn of mind. Each person has what is commonly called a "general attitude" that is cumulatively established and controls the way he thinks. While this may suit his general life very admirably, it will not fulfill the thinking needs of a specific profession, since the only purpose of a profession is to ensure that special things will be seen and that they will be seen in a special way.

Because the professional's turn of mind is habitual and represents an integrated set of attitudes, it can be called a personality pattern. But it would have to be called a professional personality pattern, since it should be professionally rather than personally evolved. It is a second personality, grafted upon the professional by his professional training and experience, and it may be quite different from his nonprofessional personality. It could of course never be completely different, since a person's general attitude constitutes a record of all the places he has been. Ultimately, one could expect that the two personality patterns would converge, and the professional would start living like one as well as working like one. However, the professional apparently does think and act differently when he assumes the role of a professional. This is easily apparent to anyone who witnesses the change in approach and demeanor that occurs when the doctor changes into his white coat or the minister into his black one.

The important thing is that the individual professional recognizes that there is a necessary turn of mind that goes with the effective practice of his profession, and that he must be alert to obtain it, to improve it, and to prevent its deterioration. Just as with his general way of mind, his professional turn of mind is not God-given and is derived, either consciously or unconsciously. Formal education will give him a background for his professional thinking, and experience will mold it for him, but neither will ensure how he can best develop and retain it. The professional turn of mind is a type of personality trait and represents a habit pattern. As such, it will change for better or for worse as time and new experience come to pass. Only persistent practice and determination ensure that the change will be for the better, and this is up to the individual professional.

Just as there is a "legal mind" or a "scientific mind," there is an administrative mind. It represents a set of attitudes that consistently influence the way the administrator's mind works—the things he thinks about and the way he thinks about them.

In practice, these attitudes are so closely interrelated that it is difficult to determine where one ends and another begins. To a large extent they reinforce each other. Also, their influence is more general than specific, and they show more of the bent of the administrator's thinking than the substance of it. For these reasons they are more accurately described as senses rather than skills of effective administration. Here, then, are 31 "senses" that make up the administrator's turn of mind, as we have recreated them from our notes of Ray Brown's lectures.

1. The Sense of Restlessness

This is one of the most important of the senses, and because it is one of the easiest to identify it can be used to show the nature of these senses and the manner in which they influence administration. Two different hospital administrators may each be equally skilled and on a par in every way except in this one. Yet the one hospital over a period of time will greatly outdistance the other in efficiency and quality of care. The difference represents in part the difference between restlessness and complacency of the administrator.

The effective administrator is never fully satisfied with how things are done, and even the best is never good enough for him. It is not a frustrated sense but an eager one, and it can be described as an administrative discontent rather than a personal one. It does not adversely affect his personal relations with other members of the organization, because they realize it is an administrative outlook rather than a personal attack. They are affected organizationally, however, and because administrative attitudes are very catching they themselves become infected with the attitude that anything can be improved. It is through the creation of such an organizational climate of always doing better that the administrator receives the payoff from his unquieted zeal for improved results.

It is hard to pin down any great amount of overt or strong action by the administrator in getting across the notion of continuous improvement. It is perhaps demonstrated more in connection with the element of time than in any other way. He tends to be impatient with progress of activities and projects and to exhibit an urge for "newness." Those around him are impressed with the fact that life is here and now, and that things must be done as other things occur. Time takes the shape of essence, and his concern for getting things done on time somehow results in a concern on the part of others for getting things done better.

2. Sense of Incompleteness

This is a matter of how much is done rather than how it is done. It is concerned with the scope of activity and represents an eagerness to grow and to expand. It is more a desire to round out and to fill out than to add dissimilar activities. It can be described best as a perpetual feeling of unfinished business on the part of the administrator who always has plans and seems always to have something cooking on the back burner ready to bring out when the time is ripe.

3. Sense of Innovation

This is a matter of the new. It is a willingness to break loose from the conventional and move into the untried. It is exhibited in the fact that these administrators are the first to install newly developed equipment and to adopt new methods and procedures. In the manufacturing field, these administrators lead in expenditures on product development and the rate of change in product engineering and design. Their willingness to change the way things are done gives the observer an impression that they see value in change itself. This notion is not too far-fetched, since it would be a way of transmitting their own sense of innovation to all levels of the organization. It would serve to keep the organization on its toes and both ready and able to adopt change and to live with it.

This sense of innovation should not be confused with high creativity. The effective administrator rarely is of an inventive mind himself. His creativity, as such, is one of recognizing and effectuating the best ideas of others. He has a green thumb for cultivating ideas but leaves it to others to breed them. There are logical reasons why the administrator should be ingenious rather than a genius. He must demonstrate common sense to those with whom he deals, and he can do this only if he sees things mostly as those around him see them. The inventors are highly creative, on the other hand, and must see things differently if they are to perceive something that has previously gone undiscovered. The administrator needs to recognize and utilize the highly creative, but he does not need to be creative himself.

There is another anomaly that needs to be reconciled in this description of the administrator as an innovator. While he is an innovator of process and product, he can be classified generally as a conservative ideologically. This apparent ambivalence has its logical explanation. First, it should be pointed out that he is not the reactionary that he is often painted to be. He is a progressive rather than a radical and is described best as conservatively progressive rather than progressively conservative. It is the legal, political, and economic rules that give him concern. Each of his decisions represents a prediction of the future that is based on the past, and it is hard enough to predict the unknowable future, without having the base changed. His interest is not one of holding onto the pastness of the past but one of maintaining a stable set of ground rules, so that he can make sense out of the past.

Admittedly, he is likely to be much more pragmatic than philosophical. He is responsible for the results, and this forces him to be more interested in producing than in preaching. Experience has disillusioned him as to the likelihood of a perfect world and has made him want to get on with the job of making the best of this one. Because he must get things done, he has to be more interested in what this world he works with has than in what it lacks, and to want to make do rather than make over the character of it. Stated another way, he believes in social progress but also believes that it is sold by the inch and therefore he has a deeply ingrained suspicion of any schemes that promise to deliver it in wholesale lots.

4. Sense of Personal Adequacy

This has to do with the level of self-confidence and self-sufficiency possessed by the administrator. The most effective administrators feel up to the task and show it. They do not see themselves as dependent on the whim and caprice of providence but believe that the door to success is locked from the inside and that they have the key. Because they trust themselves, they are unlikely to get buck fever and panic when the going gets rough. This trust is demonstrated in their ability to adjust well to frustrations, confusions, and criticisms, and their overall stability in pressure situations. Since the administrator knows his strengths, he doesn't feel he has to hide his weaknesses by going on the defensive when he happens to make a mistake. Because he believes in himself he believes in his decisions, and this permits him to be decisive. It is confidence rather than conceit, however. This means that he is not dogmatically sure of his ground, but sure of himself. It also means that he is not so full of himself that he has no room for anything else. Stated another way, he is able to be dominant without being domineering.

The self-reliant administrator has faith in himself, but it is not a blind faith. It is a responsible and measured faith that permits him to be courageous without being foolhardy. A sense of personal adequacy is not possible unless there is also an awareness of one's inadequacies and limitations. No mortal is ever totally adequate, and the self-reliant can remain that way only if they know when to seek assistance. This does not mean that the administrator will defer too much to others, but rather that he has sufficient self-confidence to permit him to delegate and let others have ideas.

5. Sense of Accountability

The administrator is not only able but is also willing to pay the price. He knows that administration is not a spectator sport, and that he must accept the risks involved. It is more than a sense of responsibility. It is that plus a feeling of being answerable. He is willing to be liable as well as responsible—to commit himself and to stake his reputation on the results. This sense is exhibited by the fact that the administrator accepts organizational problems as his own and feels a strong obligation or commitment to the job. He follows through on problems and projects and finishes what he starts. Because he takes his own work seriously, he is likely to place more stress on reliability than on creativity in evaluating his subordinates. This doesn't mean that he is opposed to the novel but rather that he does not believe in avoiding the onerous.

6. Sense of Purposefulness

The effective administrator works hard at whatever he does. He sees himself as a person who causes things to happen. He takes himself as well as his work seriously, and has a deep, basic urge to get things done. He is action oriented and wants to change things rather than just explain them. In a real sense he works hard for the sake of working. This is demonstrated in his enthusiasm for his work and in the fact that he is not easily discouraged. He exhibits determination and tenacity and a sort of "doggedness" that makes him capable of long sustained effort. Because he gets his highest satisfaction from work, there is likely to be little distinction between his work and his leisure activities. He often carries his work home with him because he likes it and not because he has to.

The fact that the effective administrator has such strong work commitments causes him to identify himself more closely with his work than with the organization. He also identifies himself more strongly with results than with goals. This raises some doubt about the commonly held notion that the administrator must believe strongly in the purposes of the enterprise in order to work hard at putting them across. It is probably true that it is difficult for him to work hard for something that he personally opposes, but this is about as far as the effect of his personal predilections seems to go. This does not mean that the effective administrator is amoral, it means that he responds more effectively to the situation before him. Sincc hc docs not have to be motivated by anything beyond the work he faces, he is largely self-motivating and self-starting.

7. Sense of Detachment

The good administrator tries to keep his psychological distance from those around him. He uses the axiom that good psychological fences make good organizational neighbors. Because he knows the penalties of getting his emotions entangled with his work and the difficulties of the administrator obligated by personal ties, he attempts to remain emotionally apart while still being a part of the organization. This does not mean he retreats from contact with people and their problems, nor does it mean he is not warmhearted. Rather, it means that he attempts to remain unemotionally involved and to pace himself emotionally. He tries to be coolheaded without being coldhearted.

To the extent that he can succeed in being both a spectator and a participant, he can better exhibit such qualities as tolerance, good humor, and fairness. By keeping his emotions on the bench, he can work with people he dislikes and tolerate ideas with which he is in personal disagreement. It permits him to see the administrative task as a game played according to the rules rather than as a personal contest. By taking care that he does not serve as either a sparring partner or a proxy for someone else's emotions, he can recognize and observe values of others without assimilating them.

8. Sense of Skepticism

This sense probably marks more than any other the difference between the novice and the seasoned administrator. It is the opposite of naive and uncritical acceptance. In a way, administration can be defined as a discipline of doubt, and the good administrator can be classified as a "doubting Thomas." He uses doubt as an examiner so as to discern between good and poor ideas and the sources of good and poor information. This is not because he is cynical or mistrusts people, but because he has learned enough administrative geometry to know that there are two sides to every question. It doesn't take much experience to teach him that the most objective individuals are still advocates, and he must allow for the art of advocacy that every person practices from the day he is born. To offset this selling effort of others, he develops the practice of mentally countering the facts as they are presented to him.

If the administrator is to have an open mind, he must have mental reservations that he does not allow others to fill. Otherwise, he will have no room for more than one point of view or more than one source of facts. Neither will he have any counterweight to use in weighing the validity and implications of what he is told. The proper function of the administrator is not to answer questions but to ask them. The sort of questions he asks helps determine the sort of administrator he is. The facts that he gets will not be very much better than the questions he asks and others answer. If administration ever gets its own coat of arms, it will be the question mark.

9. Sense of the Significant

This is a matter of putting first things first. Administration is a selective process, and the administrator performs by deciding among alternatives. In order to make such choices, the administrator must be able to discriminate. He must be able to spot the essential and to sense crucial relationships. Unless he can do this, he may be distracted by the irrelevant, the inconsequential, or the marginal. This can mean that he is taking the wrong things into account or giving the wrong weight to the right things. It may also mean that he is not directing his energies effectively. The job of the administrator is literally never done, and he must assign priorities to what he does do. Circumstances about which nothing can be done must be ruled out; things that must be done must be placed at the top of his attention table. Doing a thing well is not the same as doing the best thing.

10. Sense of Tentativeness

The only thing the administrator can ever be sure of is change. The effective administrator learns early in his career that nothing is final and nothing is perfect. He realizes that all decisions must be validated under constantly changing circumstances and that a truly monumental idea can, with changing conditions, quickly become a tombstone. He knows that one decision will in time require other decisions, and that administration is involved as much in undoing conclusions as in making them. This means that unless he is to make himself a prisoner of the present and lock himself into today's solutions, he must leave room for administrative maneuverability. To the extent possible he must provide himself a hedging area that will allow for the contingencies that are inherent in all solutions. His decisions need to be qualified so that some account may be taken of impacts not discernible in advance. He must seek to leave as many alternatives as possible open indefinitely.

11. Sense of Appropriateness

Because the practice of administration is so much an art, appropriateness is one of the core senses of administration. It is concerned with suitability, with compatibility, with what is fitting and proper. Administration is sometimes called the art of the plausible, because it depends on getting things done through other people, and things must make sense to people if they are to accept them. What the administrator does must not only be right but it must also look right. Because influencing others is a way of life for the administrator, he must develop a feel for people and their attitudes and conventions. He can't stop to figure out human nature anew every time he acts; he must practice administration by the touch system, since he has no time to use the hunt-and-peck method.

The way administration depends on people puts a premium on smooth social relations. The successful administrator demonstrates his social ability in his work. He knows the value and learns the way to associate successfully with others. He doesn't necessarily have a great liking for people, but he makes it a point to learn to relate well to others in his work.

Because the administrator is walking on psychological eggs, he must know and understand the expectations of all the groups with which he deals. For instance, if he is to be just and fair he must know what makes justice and fairness. These are not exact concepts and their definition varies by group and by geography. They are what people think is appropriate. This means the administrator must be strongly reality oriented. He looks more for compatibility than for theoretical justification in decision making. He wants reasonableness more than preciseness as a guide. He pays respect to scientific method, but may pay it little actual attention. The more complex the problem the more likely he is to use his judgment rather than any refined measurements. He knows the question of feasibility is more important than one of perfection. This means that he does the almost impossible, being imaginative in an orthodox way.

12. Sense of Propriety

This is a sense of how things ought to be done. It is a belief that everything takes place within a certain discipline and all the ends are tucked in just right. The administrator knows how things should look, and how things should be accomplished so that they will look right. He does have an attachment to tradition, formality, and decorum. He knows or is aware of those things one should change and those things that should not be changed or should be allowed to evolve.

13. Sense of Discrimination

Nearly every administrator understands the sense of discrimination as knowing that he can't put his spoon into every pot. Real discrimination means that one notices the differences between things that appear similar and the similarity among things that appear different.

The administrator demonstrates a high degree of ability to fit apparently isolated factors into a structured whole. He gets his pictures in unassembled jigsaw fashion and must put them together for himself. It really is what the administrator sees and how he sees it that determines how he will handle a situation or problem. He cannot refuse to deal with problems because their course is obscure or the facts are fuzzy. But what the administrator sees and how he sees it determines how he will handle it.

14. Sense of Perplexity

This sense has to do with an intellectual curiosity or an inquiring mind. The administrator must have an almost compulsive need to know what's going on.

But it is more than curiosity; it is a discipline of doubt. It is never believing everything that is said. For sometimes one hears half-truths, and one may be hearing the wrong half. The ability not to accept information without first looking into it critically is important. It is a profound sense of the need always to be on the horns of a dilemma, forever raising doubts and asking hard-hitting questions. The sense of perplexity is the art of asking oneself critical questions that lead either to new answers or to revitalizing.

15. Sense of Fatalism

Like all professionals, executives are not devastated by loss; they really expect to lose sometimes. The professional baseball player, who gets a hit his first time at bat and is batting 1.000, realizes he will never maintain that batting average. But it doesn't bother him. The administrator realizes that he will make mistakes, and he learns that he can't fret over mistakes; as the saying goes, he learns not to cry over spilled milk. He has an ability to get over his mistakes, to put them behind him and move on to other challenges. He doesn't worry about the past because he knows he can't escape the past, but he can change the future.

A sense of fatalism enables the administrator to recognize the consequences of organizational life; there is a high degree of probability involved. His relationship with others puts an "if" into his plans and decisions. Interdependent relationships and his own integrity dictate periodic reassessment and redirection. The failure of future events to occur according to precise specifications and precise timetables produces neither frustration nor breached relationships. He knows that few things in life are the way he wants them, and he can live with this.

In other words, he has to accept life on the terms of what life produces. If he isn't able to do this, then he's going to carry grudges; he's going to carry hostilities from one question or one problem over to another. If he's going to be fair to people, then he should let each problem stand on its own, and not carry the problem or the impressions he got from it to another problem. Obviously, he can never do this successfully, because his opinions of people are built up over a series of contacts. That's all right, if he just remembers that he should not carry these feelings as facts into the new situation. Too often, feelings are confused as facts, and the administrator judges the situation as he judges the individual rather than the situation itself.

The administration must realize that management requires a lot of trying and a lot of failing. He has to assess his own performance honestly—and that will be humbling at times. But he also knows better than to brood over problems that are patently beyond his control, and he doesn't dwell on incidents to extract the last drop of irritation. He learns the value of an occasional retreat—he has no need to just stand and suffer.

The administrator with a sense of fatalism is more interested in what he can salvage rather than in what he has lost. He attacks problems in terms of the future, and he forces them to come to him in single file. He can take substantial risks with reasonable equanimity.

16. Sense of Urbanity

This sense is the ability to demonstrate broad-mindedness or adaptability. Urbanity of mind allows the administrator to work with people he dislikes and to tolerate ideas with which he is in personal disagreement. This sense also allows him to recognize and observe the values and feelings of others without assimilating them.

The administrator with a sense of urbanity can be uncommitted to a cause he represents, and yet still be greatly concerned about representing it properly. He can become involved with ideas without real emotional or personal support for them.

Indifference to certain ideas does not legitimize dishonest or unethical behavior, but a sense of urbanity enables the administrator to take things in a "man about town" fashion.

17. Sense of Foresight

The sense of foresight enables the administrator to predict the state of events at some future point in time or year. The ability of foresight may be considered as: the ability to think of a large number of alternative events in the future; the ability to judge among scenarios as to their probability; the ability to judge as to their importance among possible consequences; the ability to decide the best course of action among all the given consequences; the ability to decide the best course of action among all the given consequences likely to follow. Foresight, then, is conceiving the future in the present.

But this sense of foresight is more than thinking ahead. It includes doing ahead. It foresees things in the sense that one sees to his chores. It not only conceives the future but seeks presently to provide for it, a bifocal vision that sees the long-term as well the short-term. There can never be much positive planning, because the future, as a concept, is almost completely restricted to an extension of present perceptions—a projection of the present reality. Our only conceptions of the future are those based on perceptions of existing phenomena.

Foresight is evaluated on the basis of what was done beforehand, judgment on what occurs afterward. The sense of foresight is more of preparedness than of performance. It is more concerned with readiness than with occurrence, or more with eventualities than with actualities.

This sense of foresight is important, because the administrator must mentally cross the bridges before he gets to them. Seeing the bridges before he gets to them as well as taking action before he crosses them is foresight.

18. Sense of Timing

A sense of timing enables the administrator to show restraint and to bide his time. He recognizes that there is a time and a place for everything, and he has the ability to wait out the situation.

The smart administrator knows that *when* he does something is as important as what he does and how he does it.

19. Sense of Relevance

It is vital for an effective administrator to distinguish what is important. The diversity and multiplicity of the administrator's world can crowd him into corners of irrelevance. Often, the sense of relevance is the difference between success and failure. An intelligent and energetic administrator can go down the tubes by dwelling on irrelevant matters.

The position of the administrator determines much of what life is about. Acquaintances, lifestyle, and even ideas and thoughts influence the feelings that are a part of his view of relevance. The administrator senses the need to recognize his own inadequacies and learns relevance the hard way.

Perhaps learning the hard way is the best, or the only effective way to learn. But learning the hard way is hard on the organization as well as on the learner. Those from whom he learns may pay the price of his learning. This payment is inescapable but it need not be so high nor so repeated.

The price of learning the hard way can be lowered if the administrator honestly recognizes those things around him that are important and does not allow himself to be led astray by those things (or people) that are not. His own sense of relevance enables him to remain focused on the purposes of the organization.

20. Sense of Nowness

Life is a very daily thing to the effective administrator. He realizes that he and his organization survive on what gets done today, and he identifies much more strongly with results than he does with long-range goals, although these goals are very important to him.

The administrator with a sense of nowness knows he cannot disengage himself, or the enterprise, from the tide of daily events. He is action-oriented; he knows that even if he is on the right track, he will get run over if he just sits and waits. Even the ablest administrator cannot fight today's wars with tomorrow's plans. He knows it is better to be present than to be perfect.

The sense of nowness causes the administrator to know that he must live in the here and now. He has to use the day at hand—he'll never have it again!

21. Sense of System

The sense of system is the ability to sense the right administrative symmetry, the ability to really see the forest and the trees, and then to see each tree and its relationship with every other tree in the forest. It is similar to the way a quarterback sees the whole field or a point guard sees the whole court and where each team member is in relationship to the sidelines and the basket.

But in addition to the system space perception, there is an equally important time perception. The administrator has the sense to see the effect of one action on the total organization as well as on each of the key members of the team. This sense enables him to categorize actions or the effects of those actions for now and for the future.

The administrator with a sense of system "can put two and two together and get four without knowing the second two." He not only recognizes when parts are missing—but he knows which parts. He sees the organization as a whole. He is intuitional, and he has a high degree of ability to unite unstructured situations. The sense of system enables the administrator to discover previously undetected relationships among facts and other considerations and to evaluate situations in their largest context.

22. Sense of History

The administrator with a sense of history recognizes that he must know and respect history if he is not to repeat the mistakes of the past. A sense of history is a sense of tradition, or realizing that the past has something to tell.

While the young administrator frequently has little feeling for history, the experienced executive draws on previous problems, events, and situations for methods to handle his current problems. He uses the "rough trail of experience" and realizes that past experiences of both successes and failures can be great teachers.

The time dimension is important to this sense; the effective administrator must be able to recognize when and where the winds of change are blowing—and how fast!

Something has preceded every event or experience, and there is always more in the background of the situation that the administrator can know. It is his recognition that this history exists that prevents him from thinking each problem is a crisis, or is unique. The administrator must have faith in the similarity and harmony of events over time.

23. Sense of Direction

A sense of direction provides the administrator with continuity and consistence that enables him to handle many highly varied activities and responsibilities at one time. He can turn quickly from one problem to another and back again without getting lost in an administrative thicket. He has a built-in administrative road map and the ability to recognize guideposts so that his direction is clear.

The effective administrator must have goals, but he cannot be too certain about where he is taking the organization. His goals will change as he reaches toward them. He constantly seeks reorientation, and he has wide and varied interests. He is a joiner who joins organizations not because he is gregarious but because he wants the opportunity to know and assess community leaders. His affiliations are more for purposes of evaluation than identification. His sense of direction enables him to see the differences between following the hounds and going on an administrative wild goose chase.

24. Sense of the Compatible

A sense of the compatible enables the administrator to recognize what will fit rather than what is fitting. He seeks reasonableness and values interrelationships. He knows what will be accepted under most circumstances, and he tries to identify and meet the expectations of various interest groups.

The administrator with a sense of compatibility will try harder to be relevant than to be right. He is never an extremist; he is willing to compromise, to accept what works. He seeks a solution that will satisfy himself and the environment. He looks for the best solution that fits rather than just the best solution.

Although he will be familiar with scientific methods of management, when faced with complex problems he relies on his own judgment rather than on refined measurements. He knows that the margin for error is often wider than the margin for time to act. He is more interested in compatibility than in theoretical justifications in decision making.

The administrator with a sense of the compatible will recognize when he is on a collision course. This enables him to proceed because (1) he realizes he is on it, and (2) he can be ready to jump off when necessary. This is keeping in tune by keeping your antennae out.

25. Sense of Feasibility

When defining a sense of feasibility, administration can be described as the art of the accomplishable. The good administrator will be sensitive to what he can do and will make decisions that can be carried out. He realizes that success comes only from accomplishments, so he understands and faces up to reality.

The effective administrator doesn't try to take more from a situation than the situation can stand, because he knows that if he does, most likely he will have to give it back—with interest. He does not want to be marked by heavy effort and light results, because results, not effort, are the bottom line. Therefore he doesn't demand more than is necessary to get the job done and satisfy the situation.

The administrator with a sense of feasibility has a strong reality orientation, and he won't waste his time on circumstances about which he can do nothing. He has learned when to stand and when to retreat.

26. Sense of Competitiveness

The effective administrator has a sense of competitiveness—he likes to compete against others, and, even more, against himself. He wants to win, so he is willing to take risks. He is aggressive; he has a strong achievement drive, and his real satisfaction comes from accomplishing things. He is determined to do every assignment better than it has been done before.

There is a danger that an administrator who is too competitive may develop questionable practices to avoid losing. Thus the executive does not allow his competitiveness to become the dominant drive for success. The effective administrator fights to win instead of fighting to avoid losing. He is spurred on rather than discouraged by adversity. He is optimistic and will believe that something can be done about anything.

In order to grow, an administrator must learn to stand up to the stress and strain of disharmony and competition. When faced with difficulty, the administrator with a sense of competitiveness is more likely to take over than to take cover.

27. Sense of Wariness

A sense of precaution causes the administrator to take chances, but he leaves little to chance. The competent administrator will take many risks, but he will also take many precautions that the less competent will overlook. He has a necessary amount of anxiety that must season every decision.

But it is concern, not dread, that characterizes an administrator with a sense of precaution. He is venturesome, but not irresponsible; he doesn't disregard consequences, but he does calculate their risks. He has a healthy suspicion. He knows that administration is one of the few games of chance where all sides can lose. He can never be certain, but he knows when to be uncertain. He walks around a problem until it is organizationally feasible to grab hold of it. He doesn't try to make foolproof decisions, but he tries not to be foolhardy.

28. Sense of Balance

The administrator with a sense of balance is a steady individual who doesn't go off on tangents and who has the ability to balance many different activities without going to pieces. He adjusts well to irritations, frustrations, confusion, and criticism; he accepts the fact that life is full of problems, and he learns to live with anxiety.

A sense of balance provides the administrator with enough administrative meteorology to enable him to discriminate between prevailing winds and intermittent breezes. He has the necessary amount of shock absorption for the inevitable bumps; he knows that something is always wrong with something. He doesn't panic.

The administrator is "like the high wire artist—either good or dead." The effective administrator walks a fine administrative line and doesn't go so far out of line that he can't jump back to the middle of the road. His perceptions and sensibilities are well disciplined so "when knocked down, he lands on his administrative feet."

29. Sense of Professional Attitude

The administrator with a sense of professional attitude is the best organizational man in the organization. He sees himself as a pro. He knows that he is part of a cast and that he, too, must follow the script that has been written for the role he is playing.

The administrator's sense of professional attitude provides him with a philosophical commitment to administration. He believes that the greatest payoff is in the solution to problems and that resolving problems and directing the organization should take precedence over his personal drives and goals. He sees himself as the most obligated individual in the organization.

The professional administrator has been schooled to respond to stimuli in specific ways. He accepts authority, and he works hard to understand his job as well as working hard at it.

30. Sense of Organizational Rhythm

The administrator with a sense of organizational rhythm can sense a developing problem or weakness in the organization. He is aware that whatever he does has consequences for the organization, and he anticipates actions of others. He is sensitive to the mood of the organization and its members.

This sense enables the administrator to know intuitively when and what kind of events are taking place in the organization. As one thing changes, it causes other things to change. Understanding the organizational rhythm enables the administrator to know how he can touch the organization in one place and cause a change in another, perhaps seemingly unrelated part. The administrator knows that the more complex an organization is, the better it may hold together; like a ball of yarn, the more tangled it is, the harder it is to pull apart.

He recognizes and uses this tangle to solidify his position and gain support for his ideas. By pulling on the right string, he can roll the organization in the direction he wants it to go.

31. Sense of Probing

The sense of probing enables the administrator to make inductive leaps, to perceive old data in new designs. This sense is reflective rather than reflexive—it is the act of turning over or probing old ideas.

The 31 senses that are discussed here are not the full catalog of tendencies that make up the administrative mind as Brown described it. There are others of major significance. Neither has this discussion examined fully and in detail the nature and implications of those that are discussed. The ones that have been discussed can at least provide some fruitful questions that the administrator may ask himself and against which he may make a comparison of his own dispositions. This can stimulate conscious development reflexes by design rather than at random.

Chapter Two

Administrative Strategies

The fact that the best laid plans of mice and men often go astray indicates that there is more to administration than has been meeting the eye in the management literature. We have developed a large body of useful knowledge on planning and decision making, but we have failed to give equal time to implementing our plans and decisions. It is as if the artist worked hard to achieve the precise mix he wanted in his colors but paid little attention to how he applied them. The decision determined the means, but administration also includes the employment of the means.

It is quite probable that the manner of employing the decision is in most instances a more important determinant of the degree of success of an administrative action than is the decision itself. It may also be the most important differentiator between the levels of accomplishment of different administrators. Many administrative decisions are ready-made by the circumstances inherent in a problem, and many others are self-evident because of the circumstances surrounding the problem. In such instances the decisions reached by different administrators would most likely be the same. Even for very complex problems, the likelihood of similar decisions by different administrators is very strong. But the level of results obtained from similar decisions varies greatly among different administrators.

Thus it is in the art of employing the means that the greatest area for variability in administrative effectiveness exists. This is the area which reflects most significantly the personal contribution of the administrator and hence reflects most clearly the differences between administrators. Doing the right thing is not the same as doing it well. One of the most important elements in determining the outcome of administrative action is conducting the action. This conducting represents the strategy used by the administrator.

The fact that there are many successful administrators is evidence that there exists some set of effective strategies that are being used in administration. Some of these are mentioned occasionally in management articles, but no specific study of strategy has been reported. The following listing and brief discussion of several strategies commonly used in administration represents some of the results of an effort to do such a study in past years. The study consisted of an attempt to identify and describe the strategies employed in various situations by colleagues in our own organizations, by executives with whom we were acquainted, and by executives whose actions were reported in newspaper stories and management journals. It is possible that those utilizing the strategies did not always realize that they were employing a specific strategy and were acting intuitively rather than from deliberate choice of strategy.

The practice of administration is in large degree an art, and it is possible to be highly effective without fully understanding or recognizing the individual components of the art. This does not mean, however, that such understanding would not be beneficial. It would reduce the time and the mistakes involved in the trial-and-error approach to acquiring the art. It would also assure greater consistency in effectiveness and permit continued improvements by conscious effort.

This list is by no means exclusive and represents only a portion of those the authors found to be commonly used. The ones included in this discussion were selected to illustrate the nature of strategy as a major component of the art of administration, and to show some of the techniques in the use of a particular strategy.

The list is concerned only with those strategies that are ethically and socially acceptable. Others were identified that violated the spirit of fair play and could be described as Machiavellian. In further explanation, some of those described here are in obvious conflict with one another. This is as it should be. Strategy is used in specific administrative situations, and different situations call for different strategies. The use of the appropriate strategy is one of the real tests of the administrator. The fact that a choice of strategy must be made, either deliberately or intuitively, and the consequences of such choice on the outcome of administrative actions, are ample reply to the prediction that mathematical formulae and computerized thinking will replace the administrator. Getting the answer to problems may become largely a science, but using the answer will always remain largely an art. The art consists mainly, if not wholly, of these 42 strategies described by Brown.

1. Timing

The strategy of timing is perhaps the most easily recognized of administrative strategies, and also the simplest to describe. It is a matter of opportuneness and is described in such axioms as "a stitch in time" and "strike while the iron is hot." Its importance is not always recognized, however. Some administrators seem willing to spend an endless amount of time in the study of a problem and the development of a solution, but show little willingness to spend even a small amount of time studying the most appropriate time to make the move in implementing the solution. Good solutions often lose much of their effectiveness because the administrator moves too soon or too late. For every solution there is a magic hour when the tide is running with the administrator, and the determination of that time by deliberate and conscious effort is as important as the solution chosen. The administrator must not only determine the proper timing, he must also observe it. This means he must learn to live with unsolved problems if he is to avoid moving prematurely. On the other hand, it means he must live with his unsolved problems very uncomfortably if he is to avoid being caught napping with them.

2. Generalization

This strategy calls for the administrator to start with as general a concept as possible in his efforts at problem solving. There is a distinct disadvantage in moving from the abstract to the specific. There are fewer chances for individuals to disagree when objectives, or solutions, are stated abstractly. As things become more specific, opinions have more opportunity to become differentiated, and hence the likelihood of opposition is correspondingly increased. For this reason, the administrator should attempt to close the matter once agreement in principle has been reached. He can take it as an administrative fact of life that when individuals already agree in principle, any attempt to define more precisely what they have agreed on is more likely to produce conflict than further accord. At the point when he first obtains general consensus, it is wise for him to accept responsibility for working out the details and later to delegate the assignment to a single individual.

3. Decisiveness

This strategy takes advantage of the age-old axiom that people follow strength. Its best use in administration is found in those instances when the decision to be implemented may be lacking in appeal, or may appear to be weak. Of course, the administration should always seek the strongest solution to a problem, but there are many times when the best possible solution is still a weak or doubtful one. Under such circumstances, the weaker the solution, the more decisive must be the manner of implementation. This does not mean that he can ever afford to four-flush or pretend the answer is a good one when it really isn't. Rather it is the best solution—but still a weak one. The strategy has the characteristics of a finesse in bridge rather than those of a bluff in poker. Said another way, the administrator cannot expect others to have more confidence in his decisions than he shows himself.

4. Ambiguity

This strategy is in a way the opposite of decisiveness. For many reasons, there are times when the administrator must utilize the administrative stall. This may be because he doesn't know what to do, or because of timing, or because he prefers to have others move first. Generally it is not so much a matter of indecision as one of withholding decision. Because he can't afford to expose his hand until he is both sure and ready, he has to avoid committing himself in any fashion. He does not attempt to deceive, but rather obscure. Because he cannot indicate which way he intends to move, he cannot encourage or discourage suggestions by others. Since most persons will infer approval if they don't get a negative response, the use of this strategy means that the administrator must take care to be poker-faced, or otherwise appear later to have been two-faced.

5. Minimizing Expectations

The administrator is constantly involved in selling his ideas and decisions to those who must carry them out. In his effort to gain support, he has a tendency to oversell and overpromise. His best strategy, however, is to minimize expectations. Disappointment is the difference between what people expected and what they got. By promising as little as possible and doing as much as possible, the administrator may be able to reserve a margin of accomplishment that represents a dividend of credit for himself. Since he is judged by what he does relative to what he was expected to do, there is no advantage in promising any more than is necessary in order to get his ideas accepted. He really gets no credit for the extra result he promises, and he can expect no green stamps for the promises he doesn't deliver. Said in other words, one way to reduce the negativeness of a situation is to increase the expectation that the situation is going to be negative. This does not mean that he should become a disciple of gloom. This characteristic would soon become recognized much as it has in the case of football coaches who have overplayed the strategy of predicting a losing season. Rather, the strategy means that the administrator must be realistic in what he leads others to expect, in order to prevent disappointment for them and discredit for himself.

6. Least Controversial Approach

This strategy recognizes the fact that people can get their backs up quicker than they can back down. It represents an attempt by the administrator to study each problem and anticipates various levels of opposition that he can expect to encounter. He then takes up first those parts on which he feels there is likely to be the least controversy. This helps maintain a climate of agreement by keeping the strongest feelings from being expressed at the start, and it also keeps opposition from accumulating. An axiom of selling is to keep the customer from saying "no." Once a person commits himself and puts his foot down, he somehow feels he loses face by moving his foot. We always attempt to justify everything we do and go to great lengths to prove that we were right. This is true even on things that would otherwise be of little concern to us. Also, we sometimes find ourselves defending a position that we got stuck with simply because of chance remarks. These tendencies of people impose on the administrator the often difficult task of getting a person to admit he has changed his mind, as well as getting him to change it.

Working from the easy side up also saves administrative time and effort in another way. If he works from the easy side, he is always facing only the easier level as he moves forward. If he makes a frontal attack instead and starts with the hard part, he may permit opposition to gain strength and persist, instead of subsiding.

7. Simplification

The use of this strategy permits the administrator to strip off the administrative underbrush that would otherwise complicate the solution of a problem. It involves the single-issue approach to a problem so as to avoid tangential issues that increase the chances of opposition. Problem discussions have a tendency to branch out and envelop other unsolved problems, even those with the remotest sort of relationship. This not only multiplies the number of persons and interests involved but also multiplies the number of problems and complicates the solution, because it will have to fit two or more problems rather than one. Killing two birds with one stone may be an admirable ambition, but if it ever occurred it would have to be classified as a freak. A *good* solution that fits two different problems is even more freakish.

This strategy can be used in reverse if the administrator wishes to delay arriving at a solution or to prolong a situation for other strategy reasons. By introducing new issues or broadening a simple issue, he can gain support against a particular solution that might be emerging contrary to his wishes. By combining issues he can succeed in combining forces against an uncommon opposition. If this does not serve to smother the idea, it may still help cancel its effect by maximizing the difficulties in implementing it and minimizing its consequences.

8. Flexibility

The administrator can use this strategy to avoid fencing himself in. It helps him recognize that all administrative decisions are tentative and contingent, and that he is perpetually being faced with problems of changing his mind and his policies. If he commits himself too tightly or makes his policies too rigid, he will not have the necessary room for administrative maneuvering when situations and circumstances change. By providing a margin for change, he can shift gears without shifting course when the going gets tough. Not only do tight agreements have a penchant for pinching the administrator's toes but they also are more likely to produce discord than to extend accord. Tight decisions, like tight fits, can cause friction in relationships.

Flexibility of decisions helps the administrator answer one of the major moral questions inherent in the administrative process. The surest thing in life is change, and the primary task of the administrator is to administer change. He adapts the organization to change by changing its policies and practices. But such changes may mean that he is letting down those who were depending on the existing policies and practices. All administrative decisions represent treaties or agreements with various elements of the internal organization and the external environment. Sometimes they represent actual trades made by the administrator. Whether implied or explicit, decisions are pacts, and people have a right to count on them. They must count on them if they are going to commit themselves fully to them and give the administrator the support he needs to put them across. Thus he is often faced with the moral dilemma of letting people down or failing in his responsibilities to the enterprise. The more flexible the position the administration maintains, the less this dilemma will plague him when change becomes necessary.

9. Shock Troops

Stated briefly, this strategy gives recognition to the fact that face-to-face discussion does not always produce solutions that fit back-to-back. It consists of having discussion and negotiations conducted by someone at a level in the administrative hierarchy lower than the person responsible for the final decision. By reserving final authority, the administrator gains several advantages. It protects a margin for further negotiation and thus holds the question open until all the facts and feelings have been fully revealed. Because the final authority is not present, proposals and counter-proposals can be examined without the pressure of final commitment. This strategy permits the top administrator to test the situation and locate the boundaries available for bargaining. If the situation is tense, the necessity to refer to the final authority permits a cooling-off opportunity. The referral strategy can also be used as a delaying action, as well as a method of wearing the opposition down.

However, the strategy has a value other than serving as an administrative holding device. We think of decisions as being logical derivatives, but they are in part social derivatives. We are "people-minded" and make decisions in terms of the people involved in the idea or the problem. Our tendency is to strive to reach agreement with persons, even strangers, when we are in direct contact with them. The use of intermediaries helps remove the administrator from the zone of personal influence and permits him to evaluate the situation more objectively.

10. Single Dose

This strategy is based on the arithmetic fact that one bad loss is better than two. There seems to be a point at which the seriousness of a loss cannot be increased by added loss. This enables the administrator, when confronted with a loss of some magnitude, to make a general write-off of other losses rather than have them show up separately over an extended period. An illustration of this one-shot strategy is seen in the actions of airplane manufacturers in recent years, when they chose to write off in a single year large losses that could have been spread over several years. By this strategy, they cleared the future by taking advantage of an immediate situation that was so bad that it couldn't be worsened.

11. Depersonalization

There are many times when the administrator wishes he were somewhere else. The depersonalization strategy helps him partly make that wish come true by divorcing him from the administrative situation. It attempts to put all parties to a problem on the sidelines and let third parties run through the script for them. A number of techniques may be used in employing the strategy. One technique is for the administrator to discuss the problem hypothetically, as if it had occurred elsewhere. Another is to use the third person pronoun when discussing persons involved and the first person plural when referring to himself: We, not I. Further efforts toward impersonalizing decisions include basing them on precedent whenever possible, and stressing the effects on the total organization. Other techniques involve having a third person present when discussing the problem and reserving final decision (even though both parties are fully aware of what it will be) for a respectful period; also making decisions known in writing instead of in person.

12. Taking Initiative

The strategy of taking the initiative calls for the administrator to beat the opposition to the punch. Like a good quarterback who stays on the offensive, the administrator calls the shots, and the opposition reacts to his game plan.

First impressions are lasting impressions. By taking an early, thoughtful position with employees, trustees and the public, the administrator leaves a difficult task for effective opposition to already established reactions. The first impression an administrator makes is most likely to be remembered.

Also, the effective administrator is always the first to announce bad news. Bad news travels fast, and the administrator takes the initiative by telling it his way, instead of being placed on the defensive by hostile questions. This strategy enables him to put the information in proper context.

The effective administrator also takes the initiative by seeking out and dealing with problems rather than waiting for them to be brought to him. An unpleasant answer quickly provided is better than delay and defensive action. Winners take the initiative and use their own game plan.

13. Obliqueness

The strategy of obliqueness enables the administrator to accomplish his own goals by tying them to popular goals of the majority. Complex organizations are often a setting that permits indirect movement toward a goal, to keep resistance from mobilizing. As a legislator may add a less popular rider to a popular bill in order to get it passed, an administrator may accomplish the objective of a key board member with his own ideas as riders.

A precedent can be established on a major issue by a key decision on a minor incident. This strategy might be called administration by detour. It may appear to take longer, but the administration can avoid failing to reach his destination because he insists on using the main highway, and finds it blocked.

14. Accent the Positive

Men seldom find agreement when finding fault. In the strategy of accenting the positive, when attempting to change a practice of rejecting a recommendation, the administrator uses as much as possible of the existing practice in a positive way by talking up the virtue of his idea rather than denouncing the other. A new administrator may not know the owner of the dog he is about to kick when announcing a policy change. So he should emphasize the benefits of the change, not attack the ideas of his predecessor. Being critical may force some staff member or board member to defend the old way by finding fault with the administrator's new one.

Efforts toward the goals of the institution can be maximized when the administrator accentuates the positive and eliminates the negative. Good salesmen know how to emphasize the known positive values of their product. Good administrators want to sell their public on the quality of their organization's product. This can best be done by accenting the positive.

15. Combining Issues

This strategy is otherwise described as the wet blanket technique. By broadening an issue until it includes unpleasant consequences, the administrator may weaken the support for a proposal he wishes to defeat. The technique is to complicate the solution other people see and maximize the difficulties posed. This is accenting the negative. By combining negative issues, the administrator is creating a situation whose answer becomes apparent without his outright negative response. But the wet blanket must be used sparingly. If the administrator uses it for numerous proposals, he will be viewed as negative, and his influence will be diminished. One of the chief reasons for perceived mediocrity in administration is overuse of the wet blanket technique.

16. Full Scale Review

This is an action that shows great responsiveness on the part of the administrator and focuses attention on resolution of a knotty problem. The number of mayors who appoint "Blue Ribbon" committees to evaluate politically troublesome problems is an example. The death of a construction worker in a sewer, the shooting death of an individual fleeing the scene of a crime, or the death of a patient who has been sent away from the hospital emergency room may all result in such committees. The Warren Commission that studied the assassination of John F. Kennedy is a well-known example.

An administrator should be prepared to take the initiative in ventilating the problem by bringing opposing sides together. This action shows concern and interest in an organized examination and exploration of the facts. Persons who participate as members of such a group tend to be more generous than individual critics.

The administrator should take the lead in calling for a consultant's report if a particular problem needs more visibility for a solution. The administrator will be seen as a part of the solution instead of part of the problem.

17. Involvement

When a person becomes involved in an activity, even though he may not strongly believe in it, he may get caught up and become engrossed by it. An effective leader may thus involve many people in both decision making and implementation. As others are drawn into the planning, support increases. This "conspired leadership" is a type of participative management.

Many effective executives have garnered community support by asking for input and advice from community leaders, who then buy into the operational and planning activities of the organization. People feel more kindly toward those they help than toward those who help them. By lining up help from various factions, an administrator may get others involved and bound by feeling ownership of his position.

18. Confirmation

We spend more time defending the record than trying to set a record. The idea behind the confirmation strategy is to put a person or group on record, making it difficult to change positions. If the commitment is in writing they are more likely to defend the record than to deliberate the alternatives. Many managers take a few minutes to dictate memos confirming discussions with department heads, for example, so that decisions will not slip back to more convenient recollections at some later date. It is vital that influential members of the board of trustees stand pat on their decisions when implementation is occurring at the operational level.

A variation of this confirmation approach is early action. In this approach, instead of a memo, action is taken using the agreement to establish the record of what was agreed. This is important if the administrator has a weak base of power and wishes to avoid the possibility of a reversal.

To confirm is to make firm or to strengthen. By sending a follow-up memo on a meeting, with copies to all the interested parties, the administrator solidifies his position and eliminates the alternatives.

19. Compromise

To put even a modest number of ideas into successful operation requires selling, negotiation and concession. Administration is the art of compromise. Compromise usually means integration, or achievement of the maximum area assent. The administrator knows there are times to conciliate and concede, so he gives on details in order to gain principles. Progress is often a matter of getting the participants to redefine what is acceptable.

The administrator must recognize that no one is always right and no one is always wrong. In human relationships, error will never be the only source of conflict between parties. The administrator needs to be tough-minded rather than bullheaded. There is a Wall Street saying that illustrates this: "Bulls and bears have a chance to win on the stock market, but a mule has none."

The administrator's objective is to achieve the best solution, and that may be done with an idea stolen from the opposition or conceived to overcome objections. Compromising on today's problem may give the administrator a goodwill margin for tomorrow's negotiation.

Even the most effective administrator will lose sometimes, and he will have to compromise frequently. In deciding not to compromise, he should fight only for what he has to have, and when he gets it, he should stop. When the administrator does give in, he should do so graciously but obviously.

In compromising, the administrator should never try to take more from a situation than can be given. The smart administrator learns to recognize the optimal point and stops there. He doesn't push beyond it, and he doesn't gloat. He takes his victory and goes home. An example from history was the legislative success of former President Lyndon Johnson. He initiated hundreds of new federal programs as he quoted from Ecclesiastes: "Come let us reason together." Great compromisers, from Henry Clay to LBJ have known that "half a loaf is better than none."

20. Fictionalization

When the administrator looks the other way and declines to recognize a situation, he may be employing a strategy called fictionalization. The administrator must develop "blind spots" at times in order to avoid formalizing an unsatisfactory situation. He cannot afford to take official notice unless he intends to respond or act. This strategy includes some "double-talk" that allows people to explore positions rather than taking positions.

Since human relations require a great deal of lubrication if they are to wear well, the administrator must, at times, give the other fellow a chance to "save face." Sometimes looking the other way is the best way to accomplish this. Thus the administrator may choose to act as though an incident didn't or won't happen, in order to avoid taking action. For example, he may ignore inappropriate behavior rather than initiating disciplinary action against the person; he may overlook the error of a subordinate in order to allow the person to save face; he may remain silent rather than point out that another's position has been proved wrong.

In George Orwell's *1984,* the government "fictionalized" any unpleasant event or person. At the University of Chicago, Ray Brown fictionalized the campus newspaper. He ignored the paper and read none of the editorials, so he did not feel compelled to respond to inaccuracies and inflammatory allegations while he was vice president of the university. This strategy may be useful as a face-saving device for one's opposition.

21. Linking the Effects with the Cause

The administrator will make unpopular decisions which will nevertheless require the support of those in the organization. By linking the effects with the cause, the administrator can increase the acceptability of the decision. This pairing enables the constituency to make sense of a decision which might not otherwise stand alone.

Hospital administrators typically use this practice when they raise room rates and other changes at the same time as salary increases to employees. It is obvious to all: the board, the medical staff, and the public, that the increased salary expenses will require increased revenue; hence, it is relatively easy to gain acceptance for rate increases at the time. Brown called this practice administrative hitchhiking, allowing one decision to ride or latch onto another.

A variation of this method is practiced when the administrator ties an unpopular move to a popular one. For example, the best time to increase prices in the employee cafeteria may be shortly after benefits, and particularly salaries, are improved.

A newly appointed administrator who has come in or been promoted above an existing administrative staff may evaluate salaries of members of the staff and make appropriate increases. The fact that he gave the increase establishes very clearly his authority over them. By using the pay increases to accomplish several objectives, the administrator is riding a borrowed horse.

22. Postdating the Action or Effect

An executive can use time to his advantage and to win acceptance for his decision by using the strategy of postdating the action or effect—the concept of using time as a buffer because something that is going to happen in the future seems less ominous than today's events. The meaning of an action to be taken in the future is obscured in the present. It is natural to be inherently optimistic, and so the view of the future usually appears brighter than it very well may turn out to be.

The effective administrator will use this optimism to gain support for his decisions today, knowing that the effects will occur tomorrow, and that is when the full impact will hit those involved. A simple example is the common practice of discussing an upcoming retirement with the employees a year before the retirement will actually occur. This is ostensibly done to allow the prospective retiree and the firm to plan for that retirement. But it also allows time for the employee to accept the inevitable retirement, when he really may not be inclined to retire.

Another example of the strategy of postdating the action or effect is announcing a salary increase that is to occur in the future. This provides months of good will with employees without requiring an actual cash outlay until sometime in the future. The effect is usually as beneficial as of it were happening immediately.

The administrator plans and negotiates continuously. When he postdates actions to be taken in the future, he gives opportunities for second thoughts to take hold. The delay allows others time to come around to a position of support as well as to develop second thoughts. Used appropriately, time can soften things that are a problem today.

23. Overexposure

Among the strategies for defeating ideas that are unacceptable is overexposure. The administrator beats the notion to death by keeping up the exposure. People become satiated by continued talk about a matter—so much that they begin to ignore it; momentum and support fade and die.

24. Co-optation

The strategy of co-optation is the process of absorbing new elements into the leadership structure in order to avert or eliminate threats to its stability. Stated another way, if you can't whip them, let them join you.

By increasing the number of persons involved, the strategy diminishes the intensity of the situation. As the number of participants increases, the persistence of individual interests and loyalties wanes, thereby reducing the force of the total. By adding diverse interests to the solution, the administrator accommodates many persons and weakens the will of each to work for his own goals.

The strategic planning process, as utilized by many organizations, is an example of this strategy in action. Many persons from the medical staff, governing board, hospital employees, and community at large may be included on various committees as part of the planning effort. Each will have special interests to serve, but the efforts of each will be diluted by the efforts of others. The result will be a solution which to some extent accommodates everyone, but completely satisfies no one with the possible exception of the hospital administrator. He has been able to dominate the process, because the inclusion of so many has had the effect of blending out the factions. Furthermore, the solution will have multiple affiliations and strong support because of the inclusion of diverse interests; the administrator has them with him instead of against him.

There is an inherent danger in this strategy, however, that the administrator will have to decide at what point he has sold himself down the river by getting too many Trojans in the horse. Like all strategies, this one can be effective to the extent that it is timely and appropriate. But an administrator should remember the fact that everybody's business is nobody's business is not always bad, and use this knowledge to advantage.

25. Clean Slate

The administrator's purpose is to arrive at the best possible result, not to win moral victories. Therefore it is to his benefit to start the solution of each new problem unencumbered by the mistakes of the past. This is the clean slate strategy. The effective administrator never brings up past unpleasant occurrences that might influence the attitude of other persons when discussing a current problem. He lets sleeping dogs lie and attempts to wipe the slate clean as each solution is arrived at, in order to save face for those involved, so that future situations will not be adversely affected.

Since it is man's nature to want to win moral victories, it is difficult for the administrator to avoid trying to prove himself right, but if he does, he may create enemies who will remember his victory achieved at their expense, and this may interfere with future decisions. Machiavelli said, "when you disarm them, you commence to offend them and show you distrust them either through cowardice or lack of confidence, and both of these opinions generate hatred against you." The smart administrator knows this and therefore practices administrative amnesty. He lets bygones be bygones. He knows he must win the war, but he will bury the hatchet after each battle. Whether he loses or wins, he must do so graciously. He should not seek unconditional surrender.

26. Leave Some Honey to the Bees

The administrator must not only live with his decisions but also live with those affected by them. Since in the future he will have to depend on those whom he has offended or alienated for support, it is to his advantage to leave some honey in a decision. Those who were opposed need a way to save face. The administrator has to live with the result. He is not like a judge who can expect the litigants to go away and leave him alone after he has made his decision. As he analyzes a situation and a potential confrontation, he should look for ways to enable the persons adversely affected by his decision to justify a change in position to themselves and others. For example, a key employee may be given an opportunity to resign rather than be fired. The result is the same: the administrator gets what he wants, but the employee also maintains his self-esteem and relationship with others in the organization.

27. Dissipate the Bitter with the Sweet

The strategy of dissipating the bitter with the sweet has two aspects. The first is the sandwich technique, which means to sandwich bad news between two more favorable events, thus dissipating bitterness. For example, in a disciplinary situation, the administrator may begin a discussion with an employee with positive comments. The employee will get the message without having his feelings hurt as much as they would have been if the criticism were given alone. Effective criticism should not be demoralizing.

Another example of this same strategy is starting with the bad news and ending with good news. To accomplish this the administrator must describe a situation or problem as worse than it actually is. If others think the situation is worse than it really is, they will be relieved when it turns out to be not as bad as they have thought. But thus overstating the situation is often risky, because it is human nature to gloss over our problems. However, handling a difficult situation in this manner enables the administrator not only to accent the positive aspects of a situation but also to gain acceptance for a negative alternative which at first was seen as undesirable but later seemed more acceptable.

28. Borrowed Halo

The strategy of the borrowed halo is the reverse use of guilt by association. When the administrator uses this strategy he lines up influential leaders in support of his position. He spends his efforts selling a few key people who can then influence others; thus he borrows their halos or status to convince others. The administrator knows it is human nature to accept someone who is an expert in one area as an expert in all areas. This principle is most evident in advertising, where prominent athletes and movie stars are used to sell all kinds of products that are completely unrelated to their areas of expertise. Their competence is assumed to carry over to any product they are promoting.

Nearly all administrators hesitate to oppose a respected member of the organization. But the smart administrator will line up the member's halo in order to gain support for his own programs. This tactic is a form of administrative name-dropping. The administrator has a project for which he needs the support of two influential persons, A and B. His assessment is that B will be the hardest to sell. So he sells A on the idea; then he asks A if he should talk with B about the project. A has to say yes, and that enables the administrator to approach B on the basis that A suggested he talk with him. He thus lines up the halos of two influential people, and the success of his project is likely, if not certain. Of course, the strategy can backfire if the administrator picks up the support of someone who is in disrepute or disfavor, which could have the effect of stalling the project, not selling it.

29. Definition

The strategy of definition is one in which the administrator pushes issues in order to test boundaries, or, said another way, to find out how far he can go. He probes the situation to find soft areas, and then asks others to define the meaning of terms so that he can either change the definition or identify negotiable soft areas. Then he can begin to work on the soft spots.

This strategy is often seen in status-carrying in an organization, when a person is given a problem to see how much he can settle by himself. A reverse of this strategy is giving an employee an opportunity to carve out or define a larger area of responsibility and authority for himself, as is sometimes done. The administrator may also smoke out the source of a problem by moving with corrective action into an area of poorly defined authority. During the process of correction, opposition may emerge, and problem areas of disagreement will also emerge.

30. Crisscrossing and Countervailing

These strategies enable the administrator to try balancing or offsetting one issue with the introduction of another. The crisscrossing strategy can be used to create cross pressures on an existing problem on which there is divided opinion. When the administrator faces considerable opposition, that could be the time to introduce a second difficult problem so as to divide the opposition. The second issue serves as a balancing mechanism; some members of the opposition to the first issue may be in favor of his position on the second issue. Generally, a person can focus on only one issue at a time, and this strategy in effect halves the opposition by creating cross pressures. Both the problems then have a better chance of success or compromise. But the crisscrossing strategy can be dangerous if the opposition becomes united on the second issue as well as the first.

A companion strategy is countervailing, or offsetting one thing by emphasizing something else, thus de-emphasizing the first issue with a countervailing idea, area, or problem.

31. Blow-Off Valve

In utilizing this strategy the administrator leaves a blow-off valve or face-saving device for the opposition. On many pieces of equipment there is a safety device, or blow-off valve, that is released under pressure. In a controversial situation, the administrator should thus leave a graceful way out for an opponent, especially when a loss will be obvious to others, so that the loss will not appear devastating. The effective executive always leaves a way out or permits his opponent to save face.

This strategy is commonly used in labor negotiations, where either management or labor may leave the other side a way to retreat gracefully so they do not lose face with constituents. The 1981 Air Traffic Controller Strike against the government is a good example where neither side had a blow-off valve, while in the 1981 baseball player's strike there was a blow-off valve for the owners. An administrator should never cut off the opponent's means of retreat or way out unless he is prepared for a more intense battle on the blow-off itself, or another issue. A devastating loss is never forgotten. Generals of ancient Greek armies make it a point not to cut off the enemy's retreat because they knew that if bottled up, the enemy would fight even more desperately.

In *The Red Badge of Courage*, Stephen Crane wrote, "It is not well to back men into corners; at those times they all develop teeth and claws." The effective administrator should be willing to let an opponent save face and have some glory, as long as the administrator gets what he wants.

32. Lose Big

No one wants to lose a contest or fail at something he is trying to accomplish. However, when a loss or mistake is obvious, the administrator should lose graciously. The administrator should be the first to let others in the organization know he has made the mistake, and lose big. If President Nixon had admitted his error in judgment in the Watergate break-in, he might have finished his second term as President honorably.

Administrators should be willing to admit that they are wrong. Often others are impressed with a person who can openly admit he is wrong or made a mistake. No one is perfect. Moreover, when defeat or loss is admitted, the opposition has nothing to fight and may feel good or become overconfident. Making excuses for a loss may detract from the winner's victory, but more importantly, it gives the administrator a sour grapes label and may hurt him in future conflicts.

Thus the administrator must learn to lose graciously and obviously. By doing so he will gain points with the winners, which will help him in the next contest. When defeat is certain or inevitable, the administrator benefits by being the first to admit it. He learns to make lemonade out of the lemons.

33. Turn the Other Cheek

The use of this strategy can best be understood when the administrator has made a mistake, and then makes a new proposal on the heels of a defeat. Few members of the opposition will slap the other cheek or try giving the administrator another black eye, once he has had a setback. The administrator is turning the other cheek to exploit a defeat.

The strategy of latching a new proposal or request onto defeat can be illustrated best when dealing with a regulatory agency. Once the first proposal has been defeated, the administrator should be ready to propose an alternative plan. This new plan, while slightly less ambitious than the first request, will often be accepted because people will not try to defeat him a second time.

34. Toe in the Water, or Trial Balloon

This strategy recognizes the fact that it's best to stick a toe in the water to test its temperature before diving in. The administrator can use this strategy by making a partial move toward an objective before making a full commitment. An administrator should be venturesome but not foolhardy. In the hospital, the administrator should identify several key opinion leaders on whom he can test ideas. If they go for an idea, most likely he can gain the support of the entire organization. But since their opposition would almost certainly mean failure, the administrator should not propose items they all oppose. He should find out where they stand.

Another way to put a toe in the water is to leak some information to observe the reaction. The administrator may even have a point man test the wind with a portion of it before he suggests the full proposal. By sending up the trial balloon, the administrator learns where the opposition is and what they think, and what the positive arguments may be. The strategy provides an opportunity to withdraw or change course, or to proceed in the same or a different direction based on the reaction to the trial balloon.

35. Quit When You're Ahead

When the successful administrator has won, he doesn't stand around and gloat over the victory; he takes his victory and goes home. The smart administrator knows how to stop when he is ahead. He learns that when he has made his point, additional discussion will more often hurt his position than help it. He should not overburden the golden goose. But he should recognize when he is falling behind, and stop. When a discussion ceases to be fruitful, he should postpone any further discussion or consideration, taking action to avoid stalemate. Knowing how to stop when he is ahead is a sensitivity to others that is usually developed after the administrator has gone too far several times. The good administrator soon realizes when enough is enough.

36. Decoy or Red Herring

The administrator can use this strategy by distracting attention from important parts of a proposal and attracting attention to irrelevant, less important parts. He is not attempting to hide anything, but trying continually to keep the opposition off guard by getting them to focus on relatively minor points and away from the more critical aspects of a proposal.

The strategy may be used effectively on a crucial proposal to a regulatory agency. The administrator may place several decoys in the proposal so that the review committee has several items to delete from the project in order to fulfill their feeling that they have done a good job. The administrator may also use this strategy with government surveyors by having some obvious red herring for them to spot; they may spend more time on this item and less on a more significant area. Military men use the decoy strategy by trying to get enemy forces to believe that the major thrust of an attack is coming from the right flank. The enemy reacts by throwing its reserves into the right flank, when the real attack comes from the left flank. A thorough knowledge of where the opposition is coming from is required for the red-herring strategy to be effective.

37. Hidden Hand

This strategy recognizes the fact that administrators are often considered suspect by employees. The administrator may be his own worst enemy. He may be more successful in implementing his ideas if the ideas do not appear to come from him. The use of the hidden hand strategy consists of planting ideas in the minds of others, so they can be spokesmen, sometimes unknowingly, for his ideas. The administrator can agree with someone else's suggestion and not always be the one to suggest new ideas.

The strategy may be used most effectively in dealing with physicians. The administrator should select a leader or leaders from the medical staff and plant an idea there. This takes skill and patience, and he must not appear too anxious for the physician to take the idea and run with it. If the physician is in favor of the change, with prodding he will bring it to others' attention.

Thus an important idea appears to come from a physician, not from the administrator.

38. Move from Strength

The strategy of moving from strength recognizes that once a snowball is moving downhill, it may very well be impossible to stop it—just what is hoped for. This is keeping the momentum going. The administrator should push his toughest projects when his moon is high—that is, after a series of successful ventures. The successes of the past may then carry a weaker or more difficult proposal after them in a snowball effect. Nothing succeeds like success or, in another vernacular, when you're hot, you're hot.

This strategy has been illustrated many times when a new administrator has succeeded on numerous small projects, gained the support and confidence of the board of trustees, and moved immediately into a major, high-risk venture. The smart administrator knows that everyone wants to be a winner or to back a winner. This strategy of moving from strengths is closely related to the power of positive action. Successes are positive actions, and once the momentum is going successfully, the administrator should stay on the offensive and not be distracted by what the competition is doing but devote his efforts to keeping the positive momentum.

39. Concentration of Effort

Too many balls in the air at one time is the mark of a juggler, not an administrator. Any effective executive is able to make the most of his time by attending to high priority items. Effective general managers concentrate their work and the work of their organizations on a small number of major tasks. This is similar to the so-called Prado Law or the 80/20 Rule. Eighty percent of the organization's results are represented by 20 percent of the effort.

The danger is that past successes may coax the administrator into taking on too much. The solution to a problem can be directly linked to using enough appropriate resources; a solution can be lost if the problem is tackled at the wrong time. The administrator must use the resources available where they count the most and be wary of spreading himself and his resources too thin. He must work hardest to convince those who will have the greatest influence on a decision. An experienced executive is successful largely because of his ability to keep his efforts focused on the most important things.

40. Rabbit in the Briar Patch

This classical strategy is well represented by the Joel Chandler Harris story that described Br'er Rabbit begging Br'er Bear and Br'er Fox not to throw him in the briar patch, which was in fact his favorite place to be. There is something about human nature that causes man to seek the security of his home territory. It is a well known fact in basketball that moving the game to the home court gives a significant advantage. It is worth a lot of points to have local support and the stimulus of a home environment. The administrator chooses to hold a particular meeting in his own office because he needs the familiarity and psychological advantages it provides, as opposed to the unfamiliar office of another person. The administrator should recognize the benefits of this strategy when he moves the game, or meeting, to his own briar patch.

41. Closed Doors

If the executive expects to change the mind of the opposition, he must attempt to do so without an audience. An employee does not respond well to counseling if there are others present. This cardinal rule is often violated by the same administrator who may publicly attack the ideas of someone else in the organization. The administrator should settle differences with opponents behind closed doors, and make every effort to prevent confrontation in an open forum such as an executive committee meeting. If he forces an opponent to play to an audience, he will have to maintain and defend his position, or appear to be weak in front of his colleagues. This can never bring about re-evaluation of a position in an objective way.

42. Provide Multiple Options and Alternatives

The administrator uses this strategy to avoid appearing arbitrary or dictatorial. He may offer multiple options to his staff or board, but he can select unlikely options that will not be accepted. This enables him to appear more objective than he would with a single choice. Or he may take two or more competing proposals to his governing board in such a way that the board chooses the preferred alternative. There are times when a group needs to focus on which alternative to use, instead of only on a yes or no action.

As stated earlier, the several strategies that have been described here are only a few of those identified as being commonly used by effective administrators. They are supposed to be illustrative of the concepts and are not intended to be representative of all the different situations that call for different strategies. Every situation calls for a particular strategy, as every lie of the golfer's ball calls for a particular club. To carry the analogy further, the selection of the appropriate strategy, like the selection of the proper club, is as important as the skill with which one uses it. Both are essential parts of the art of administration, and the art is the thing that helps differentiate one administrator from another.

As in the earlier illustration of what Ray Brown meant by the administrative sense of "turn of mind," the administrative strategies he described, as we have summarized them here from our notes of his lectures, are illustrated with Ray's always inventive and realistic examples based on his own experience as an administrator, and his knowledge of what works, and what doesn't.

CHAPTER THREE

FAVORITE BROWNISMS

Webster's Ninth New Collegiate Dictionary has defined an epigram as a statement that is terse, witty and pointed. Ray Brown's lectures, papers, and other published writings are rich in this kind of encapsulated wisdom, which have been called Brownisms. The few examples here have been chosen as merely representative. For anything like a full appreciation of the richness of the mother lode, readers have recourse to the originals listed in the Brown bibliography at the conclusion of this volume. The reader can pick any title at random and—as long as it has something to do with hospital administration or administrative behavior—he'll find Brownisms. Here are some of the favorites of Blanks, Corley, and Smith.

On Dealing with Change

- Changing conditions may cause a monumental idea to become a tombstone.
- When the winds of change are blowing, it is necessary to know which way and how fast.
- It is necessary to distinguish between prevailing winds and intermittent breezes.

- Knowing where you are doesn't tell you where you ought to be.
- Judgment based only on facts may be viewing the future through a rear view mirror.
- Plans for tomorrow may be fine, but there is no tomorrow without surviving today.
- The only way to get in the game is to come out of the locker room.

On Protecting your Flanks

- Before you kick the dog, find out the name of its master.
- A way to keep from striking out is never to go to bat.
- Good administration is not making the fewest mistakes but having the fewest mistakes going at the same time.
- The administrator making complex plans may risk defeat by getting too many Trojans in the horse.
- If the administrator has enough facts, the problem shouldn't come to him.
- The administrator can't sit on the summit without being on the brink of an abyss.

On the Decision Making Process

- The administrator may have to put two and two together and get four without knowing the second two.
- Face to face discussion doesn't always produce solutions that fit back to back.
- Feelings are the common cause of failing.

On Management Style

- You can't keep your eyes on the hills when your nose is on the grindstone.
- Administration is not a game of solitaire.
- Fear of losing can take the joy out of winning.

- Cold logic may melt quickly in the warm glow of friendly talk or the hot glare of opposition.
- The administrator may have to stay out of the way in order to get his way.
- The person who walks alone has to lean on himself.
- The administrator must be adept at adapting.
- The perfectionist often reaps imperfection.
- What you can get people to do is the best thing you can do for people.
- The administrator riding his hobby horse may be going the wrong way.
- The administrator has to be on hand—and learn to keep his hands off.
- The person with a one-track mind may be off course.
- To know what is going on without taking over, the administrator must put his nose in and keep his hands out.
- Improvements are sold by the inch rather than the yard.
- If the administration had a coat of arms, it would be a question mark.

On Pragmatic Considerations

- It is important to see the difference between things that appear similar and similarity among things that appear different.
- When the door to success is locked from the inside, the winner is the one with the key.
- Good psychological fences make good organizational neighbors.
- Doing something may be confused with getting something done.
- A complex organization holds together; like a tangled ball of yarn, it is hard to pull apart.

- Constantly succeeding doesn't always result in continued success.
- Trial by fire seasons the administrator, but it may result in burns and leave scars.
- Perfection is a guide, not a destination; like the North Star, it shows the way but is not the place to go.
- The best bargain may be found somewhere between selling out too soon and shelling out too much.
- The misfit may have to ship out if he won't shape up.
- It is possible to take a chance but leave little to change.
- Shooting fish in a barrel may not be sporting, but if the purpose is to get fish, it works.
- A steady diet of eating crow doesn't build strength.

On Behavioral Realities

- There is no easy way to dress up someone's performance without dressing him down.
- A person need not be kind or generous in order to act kindly or generously when it is called for.
- Behavior at times may depend more on circumstances than character, but more often it is the other way around.
- A person doesn't learn to choose a good alternative without choosing a few bad ones.
- Workouts build more strength than handouts.
- Holding the boss's hand doesn't provide as much security as toeing the line.
- The effort to make life a fiesta may create a fiasco.
- A good jockey doesn't ride a dead horse.
- People get their backs up quicker than they back down.
- In human relations, you get your change back in the same currency you pay.

Part Two

Ray E. Brown: The Doer

Introduction

David M. Kinzer

This book had its genesis in the wishes of three of Ray Brown's former Duke University students to get into published form some lectures that Ray didn't have the time to publish. It was soon apparent, though, that this one perspective couldn't do justice to Ray's contribution to the field as a teacher. There was also teaching at the University of Chicago, Northwestern University, and even a little bit at Harvard.

Beyond this, it would clearly have been a mistake to consider Ray's teaching contributions as something that could be confined to academic settings. In the view of many, his most important teaching was directed at his peers through his writing, speechmaking, and association activities, or at his subordinates in workplace settings.

It has been argued that a lot of Ray's success as a manager is attributable to his skills as a teacher of the people who worked for him or with him. One of his former lieutenants in management, Richard Wittrup, contends in the following pages that Ray was a much better teacher than a manager. But it can be argued that teaching skills are, among other things, what separate the ordinary from the excellent in management. Just to be exposed to his lively intellect with its always questioning agnosticism was an educational experience. There are a great many people still active in health care who have benefited from that experience.

So it was decided that this volume needed a Part Two and that we should invite the input of others who couldn't be categorized as only his former students. The selection process was a little difficult because there were many people still active in this category, most of them glad to contribute.

Beyond covering our bases on Ray as an educator and Ray as a manager, there was also the Ray who gave top-level political leadership to the hospital field. In fact, he can be classified as the last of the triple threats in the health care management world, perhaps the last one we will have.

There was also Ray as kingmaker. He had attained a level of influence that permitted him to give direction to the careers of numerous other leaders in the field. The field was somewhat inert politically before Ray Brown got us involved in major public policy decisions in the 1960s, especially those concerning Medicare and Medicaid. In our currently highly politicized environment, many of those now still heavily involved owe much to Ray Brown's teaching for their career advancement.

As it turned out, the inputs we chose to use in Part Two cover very well the political/kingmaker part of Ray along with the manager/teacher part. It all mixes together with surprising ease.

CHAPTER FOUR

RAY E. BROWN
PROTOTYPE HOSPITAL ADMINISTRATOR

Aaron Cohodes

The following article appeared in The Modern Hospital *in 1962, when Ray Brown had been at the University of Chicago for eighteen years in charge of university hospitals, and had spent the last year as vice president and chief business executive of the university. As it turned out, he didn't particularly like the latter job, because as he told a friend at the time, he spent most of his days buying and selling apartment buildings on property adjacent to the expanding campus. The author of the article, Aaron Cohodes, was managing editor of* The Modern Hospital. *Later, he became founder and president of Teach'em, Inc., an educational service, and a related publishing company, Bonus Books, specializing in educational, medical and sports publications.*

—Editors

As superintendent of the University of Chicago Clinics for sixteen years, Ray Brown uniquely circled his field.

He is the only graduate of a formal program in hospital administration ever to be chosen president (1955–1956) of the American Hospital Association.

He is the only course graduate ever named president of another national organization important to hospital executives: the American College of Hospital Administrators (1959–1960).

He is the only administrator from the hospital field to win the annual article award of the College, and he has done this twice (1960, 1961).

At 48, Brown is forceful, thorough, tough and a devoted friend of sweet reason. "What has made him so successful in hospital and university administration," says Dr. Lowell T. Coggeshall, vice president of the University of Chicago and Brown's long-time boss, "is his extraordinary reservoir of good solid information. He knows his facts and doesn't talk, think or act on supposed data."

Highly organized, Brown is known for practicing as an administrator what he theorizes as a teacher. His associates agree he possesses an unusual ability to distill problems to their essence, and then adduce the pertinent facts. "He dwarfs problems," says a colleague, "with his fund of knowledge."

Brown's administrative style relies heavily on ideas and issues rather than on personalities. Individuals rarely move him; concepts often do. "The personal attributes of an administrator are a bunch of baloney," he says. The effective administrator works outside them, according to Brown, and puts on special faces for special problems that have nothing to do with how he feels as an individual.

Brown credits one man with having profoundly influenced his administrative philosophy: Norman Mitchell, a University of Chicago business school professor who is now a management consultant. It was Mitchell, Brown admits, who taught him to think of management as a process, and realize that "you can get along with sorry administrative tools if you're a good artist in management."

The professional administrator, in Brown's view, is firm, logical and persuasive—and always, always, well disciplined and impersonal.

These traits are recognizable in Brown's writing, which has

won him acclaim. As a writer, Brown is what editors call a "bleeder." He works slowly, in longhand, usually carrying his ideas forward in short, fully elucidated steps that rely on Aristotelian logic to pull the reader along. He constantly revises, adding analogies, changing transitions, tightening examples—driving editors to the wall in the process by ignoring commitments and missing deadlines.

One mark of his considerable success as a writer is that the strain and agony of these revisions rarely show in print. Other shortcomings, however, do. Brown frequently repeats himself. Some of his more obvious points, such as the administrator must use good judgment, are stated and restated in his articles until they resemble a Bach fugue.

He also handles unsupportable assertions as if they were gospel. "Men like to be treated fairly," he has written, readying the reader for a disputable generality, "but they demand that they be treated impersonally."

For the most part, however, Brown impresses as well as informs, especially when he writes on his pet subject, administration. "Administration by tantrum," he has observed, "is effective only so long as the tantrum represents a change of pace." Or, returning to a familiar Brown theme: "Personal relationships represent one of the most effective sets of mind-cuffs the administrator can wear. The more intimate the relationship, the more serious is its restraint on the exercise of good judgment."

Although he is widely known as the author of a perceptive series of frequently quoted articles on administrative judgment, Brown made perhaps his biggest journalistic splash in 1956 with a paper in *Hospitals* on "The Nature of Hospital Costs."

At the time, hospital administrators were drawing heavy fire from all sides for what appeared to be an unexplainable paradox. Amid great fanfare and promises of greater efficiency and reduced costs, methods improvement men were swarming around hospitals. Shiny new equipment and technics appeared in every department to simplify and accelerate the preparation of food, bills and pills. As these measures were heralded, and the public ponied up the money to pay for them, one distressing fact kept getting in the way. Instead of dipping or even leveling, as some administrators had predicted and many had hoped, expenses climbed.

Sure, Ray Brown calmly wrote. They're going to rise indefinitely at a rate of 5 per cent or more each year. Then, in precise, reassuring terms, Brown explained why. Salaries are climbing outside the health field, and hospitals must keep pace, he noted. Industry is able to cushion much of the expense of higher wages by increased productivity, he pointed out. Hospitals can't. Because hospitals provide a personal service, he wrote, the number of hands to care for each patient simply cannot be sharply reduced, even with automation, if patient care—the end product of hospitals—is not to suffer.

This simply stated but soundly supported proposition became a battle cry for administrators everywhere. All over the country, before Kiwanis, Elks, Moose, Rotarians, Chambers of Commerce, Goodfellows, Oddfellows, Masons and the Knights of Columbus and of Pythias, administrators straightened their backs and told the bad news. Hospital costs are going to rise, they said, and they're going to continue to rise.

To their surprise, no one fainted; no one was lynched. Given a rational explanation of an inevitable phenomenon, the public reacted as it often does when it learns the worst: It sighed, then went about its business.

Brown's statement on hospital costs did considerably more than capture the imagination of the public, press and health field. By displaying the administrator as an expert on hospital economics, it served as much as any single document to strengthen the argument for lay participation in medical administration. The statement now occupies a definitive place in the literature, where it enjoys nearly as many citations as the ubiquitous Hawthorne Plant experiment of the Western Electric Co.

If writing comes hard to Brown, and it does, public speaking comes harder. Once again, it rarely shows.

"Ray sometimes puts the verb in the wrong place," a colleague observed, "but he speaks clearly and with the kind of humility and good sense that leaves listeners impressed."

Brown averages 50 speeches a year, gets butterflies each time. He never reads a speech, seldom has more than a few notes. Although his oral presentations lack the polish and thoroughness of his written work, he extemporizes with surprisingly little stammering or duplication. As a speaker, the Brown blend of country boy and university professor comes through vividly. His talks are studded with classroom words like "causative" and "conceptual" next to such colloquialisms as "you all" or "like" used for "as."

Wherever he speaks, Brown tries to say something useful and new. He often succeeds. "One thing about Ray," acknowledged a veteran science writer, "he not only participates, he contributes."

Not everybody concurs. "He's a so-so speaker," said one hospital official who has shared the platform with him several times. "Most of the time, half the people don't know what he's talking about."

On the podium, Brown likes to describe himself as a Southern Democrat. Offstage, he classifies himself as a classical economist who believes in letting society work out its own problems, as compared with Keynesian economists, such as John Galbraith and Arthur Schlesinger, Jr., of the Kennedy administration, who are more inclined to encourage government aid as a solution to social problems.

Brown, however, is less fearful of government intervention in health affairs than are most administrators. He has gone on record as favoring some sort of federal aid for the aged, taking the position that the voluntary approach has proved inadequate in this area.

This has led to criticism from conservative hospital leaders. "Brown weakens in the pressure of events and adjusts too readily to what he considers inevitable circumstances," said one of them. "He tends to adopt these adjustments as ideal objectives not only for himself to follow but for all others to follow."

Born in Union, S.C., Brown carried part of the South along with him in the form of a Carolinian twang and a tendency to give corn pone pronunciation to words by sluffing syllables (asso-say-shun) or by hitting the first syllable hard on words like hotel. Brown cheerfully acknowledges his accent, claims that neither the South nor the North can understand him, and lets it go at that.

In high school, Brown was more athlete than scholar, playing on championship teams in football and basketball. Although he describes his high school record as "miserable," Brown received from the magazine, *Scholastic*, his first national literary award for the best high school editorial of the year.

Born third from the top, Brown spent his early life hopping among the smaller towns near Shelby, N.C., with his four brothers, three sisters, and parents.

"My father," he explains, "was a Baptist minister. They have about as short a tenure as hospital administrators, both through no fault of their own."

Before college, Brown parleyed his skill as a football end into a two-year scholarship at a boys' preparatory school in Boiling Springs, N.C. In 1934, in the middle of the depression, he was ready to start at the University of North Carolina. Money was a problem, he recalls, "and my father and I had a heart-to-heart talk with the result that I started in studying as soon as I entered, and I never let up."

He received his B.S. degree from the university in 1937 as a Phi Beta Kappa. It is typical of Brown that he obtained his top grades for a clearly defined, uncluttered purpose. "Sure I knocked off those A's," Brown says. "If there's something to be handed out, the top students get it."

In Brown's case, what was handed out was a good paying job as a trust fund accountant handling endowments for the university. With this part-time job and a scholarship, he sailed through college at a small profit.

While a student, Brown took his first full-time job in the summer of 1936 in a cannery supported by the Tennessee Valley Authority. Although he was hired as an accountant, the job turned out to be as manager of the cannery. Right away, he says, "I saw I'd rather do that than be an accountant."

After graduation, Brown was soon appointed county auditor of Cleveland County, N.C., a position roughly similar to that of a city manager. He handled the budget and supervised all county functions, including the sheriff's office.

To no one's surprise, the young accountant turned in an outstanding job.

In his second year as county auditor, Brown was selected as the community's citizen of the year. In his third year, a three-way dispute among doctors-administrator-trustees at Shelby Hospital found delegates from the board and medical staff urging him to run the institution.

Flattered by the attention, Brown took a look. In 1937, after graduation, he had married Mary Witherspoon, a student at the University of North Carolina getting ready for a career in teaching.

Now, three years later, he had a daughter, and it was time to assess the future cautiously. Hospital administration, he saw, was a relatively new field with a rich potential. But there was a bug: He knew nothing about hospitals or medicine. He was reassured, however, by Dr. Watson S. Rankin, who at the time was head of the Duke Endowment Foundation. "You don't have to know medicine to manage a hospital," Dr. Rankin told Brown. "You have to know administration."

As a professional manager Brown welcomed a chance to show what he could do in a tough administrative situation. Then too, it looked as if rural city management led to a dead end. The other alternative was politics, and this seemed a gamble, even with the friendship and support of the governor and the state's two senators.

In his three years as superintendent of Shelby Hospital, Brown quickly smoothed ruffled feathers, helped build a new wing. "I didn't try to second guess the medical staff," he explains.

"When I had to criticize a physician," he says, "I did it on the basis of his relationship with other physicians, permitting him to change his mind or habits without letting the rest of the staff know."

Failure to use the medical staff organization impersonally, Brown strongly believes, is an administrative shortcoming.

"Doctors may feel they've been mistreated," he argues, "but if the affair has been handled properly, they'll feel that the mistreatment was impersonal and they will not take offense."

After three relatively uneventful years as a hospital administrator, Brown attended a two-week institute at the University of Chicago in early October 1942. As Brown tells it, "Charles Rovetta, dean of students in the school of business and head of International House, heard my Southern accent and said a fellowship of some consequence might be available if I could come back within the month."

For Brown, then 29, the prospects were unmistakably clear. He and his wife Mary never hesitated. "We sold the house and the car," he says, "and took off."

At the university, one B marred Brown's straight A record in the hospital administration program. The B, which was in Brown's specialty, managerial economics, represents, he says with a rather forced smile, "some philosophical differences between professor and student."

Brown's classmates, three men, four women, recall with awe Brown's performance as a student. "He could easily give you an inferiority complex," says Joe Friedheim, now Director of Jameson Memorial Hospital, New Castle, PA. "We used to get together and try to anticipate the questions of the instructors. Invariably, we found that if we could answer the questions raised by Ray, the examinations were easy."

"You couldn't help but be impressed with a man with one child and another on the way who was willing to give up the security of a good job and come to Chicago on a new venture," according to another classmate, Lad Grapski, director of the University of Maryland Hospital.

While a student, Brown began the process of establishing himself as a first-rate writer on hospital administration. In 1943, he published several articles on the concept of authority, relying, as he still does, on specific examples, such as the polishing of hospital silver, to keep his theoretical discussions firmly based in hospital practice.

Brown's first job with his M.H.A. degree was in 1943 as a superintendent of North Carolina Baptist Hospital, Winston-Salem. The hospital, under his direction, expanded from fewer than 100 beds to 340 beds to accommodate the newly opened four-year medical school at Wake Forest.

By the end of his first year, nibbles from the University of Chicago had started. At the invitation and expense of the university, he returned to Chicago and among others, talked with the dean of the division of biological sciences, Wendell Harrison, with Robert Hutchins, chancellor of the university, and with Dr. Arthur C. Bachmeyer, superintendent of the University Clinics.

In 1944, Brown was formally offered the position of superintendent of the University of Chicago Clinics.

For Brown, a lifelong Southerner, the move to the North was no problem. "I have always looked upon hospital administration as a profession," he says, "To me, a professional doesn't raise the question of geography or climate if he is going to be fair to his career."

Brown accepted. Reid Holmes was appointed his successor at N.C. Baptist Hospital and, on September 1, Brown was at the Clinics.

The first few months were spent on special research projects, and in early 1945 he took over as superintendent.

He promptly stood the hospital on its head. "You can call sloppy business practices humanitarianism if you wish,"said one veteran Clinics employee, "but the fact is the morale of the doctors and staff here picked up like mad when Ray started running the Clinics like a business."

Brown steadily whittled away at an annual deficit of $1.5 million until, in 1953, free of depression-incurred debts and supported by a rising economy and paying patients, the 733 bed hospital became self-supporting, and has remained so every year since.

Although Brown is well known for going by the facts, those who have seen him function in an administrative setting are equally impressed with his unusual sensitivity to ersatz ideas, a quality that enables him to recognize the worthwhile and reject the useless.

"Brown knows," says Dr. Coggeshall, "that a good plan in the wrong place is no plan at all. He's never content to accept the best of existing organizational patterns, but has a strong research motivation to go on from there."

Assistants quickly learn to approach Brown well fortified with facts. "When you come to him with a problem," said one of them, "you had better understand not only the problem, but two or three possible solutions—with all the facts to back them up. If you're basing your case on an unproved assumption—look out."

Brown prefers to handle difficult solutions himself. When a misplaced decimal point slipped through undetected, for example, unit costs of a new procedure turned out to be wildly out of line.

"We've accepted this as our decision," he snapped, with a baleful look at the assistant who had goofed, "and we'll stay with it until we can work it out."

Although he is demanding and uncompromising on quality, Brown is no martinet.

"The guy is not inhuman," said one of his students, a little doubtfully, "he's just logical as hell with a passion for getting things right."

Some indication of the respect, loyalty and affection that are felt for Ray Brown by his associates is the fact that it is virtually impossible—even under goading and promises of anonymity—to get any of them to criticize Brown in a substantive way.

"Ray knows that social recognition of employees is important," says an instructor in the hospital administration program. "He never misses an employee party. He's sympathetic to the personal problems of employees—but he's concerned without being sentimental or sloppy about it."

Brown's formidable personality and distinctive style lend themselves to imitation, and a large group of his followers, both students and assistants, have affected the Brown way of smoking a cigarette (all the way down), writing an article, and participating wholeheartedly in association activities.

The Brown penchant for work has also rubbed off on many of his associates, although not necessarily all of them.

Soon after he was on the job in Chicago, Brown started coming in unofficially on Saturday. Assistants quickly got the idea, and attendance was suddenly remarkably good in the administrative offices six days a week.

On Saturday, Brown would often assemble some of his staff and barrel into a problem by saying optimistically, "I think we can settle this in 20 minutes."

As usually happens, the minutes expanded into hours. "Who works as hard as Ray Brown—and who wants to?" complained one former assistant after an all-day Saturday session.

For the most part, however, men who have worked for Brown agree that the experience was worthwhile and memorable.

"You don't grow working for Ray Brown," said one of his associates, "you get stretched."

A typical Brown working day starts at nine in the morning.

After a day of calls, conferences and interviews, he tapers off with 90 minutes of solid dictation. At 6:30, he leaves his office, makes the five minute drive or 20 minute walk to his second floor apartment in Chicago's Hyde Park area. There he eats, generally in a gently formal fashion, with his wife and those of his three daughters who are at home. (His oldest daughter, Margaret, married to a student in the University of Chicago business school, recently gave birth to her first child, a daughter; Mary, next oldest, is a student at Drake University; Barbara, the youngest, is in high school.)

At about nine o'clock, Brown retires to his study, which has two walls completely devoted to books, floor to ceiling. Here he reads, thinks, and writes for three or four hours. In his study, Brown has assembled perhaps the best private library of medical economics literature in the country. Some 400 books, carefully indexed, touch all aspects of the subject, with emphasis on costs. Brown reads and collects everything he can on management of health institutions and he has also gathered 400 to 500 additional books on the general subject of management.

The book that through the years has influenced him most is "The Functions of the Executive," by Chester Barnard, which Brown calls "the first—and almost the last—book in which someone examines the personal contributions that the administrator makes to the administrative situation."

Brown regrets that most of his reading now must be for a purpose; he has not read fiction for 10 years, for example, and finds it difficult to make time for books that attract him intellectually rather than professionally.

In recent years, Brown has taken to playing the stock market in a modest way. Like any good investor, he reads the Wall Street Journal, Barrons, the Value line investment survey, and the evening paper (front page, sports page, financial page).

"Blue chips are overpriced," says Economist Brown. "You've got a better chance to get a ride on the unlisted stocks. Unfortunately," he admits, grinning, "I do a lot more reading and talking about stocks than buying."

As director of the University of Chicago graduate program in hospital administration since 1951, and as a full professor, Brown enjoys lecturing, follows the performance of his "boys" closely, and often helps them find a job or get out of a tight spot.

He has been closely identified with the American College of Hospital Administrators, but is able to assess it with some detachment.

"No one can be satisfied that the College has approached its potential as a professional society for hospital administrators," he says, "but the profession itself is just emerging. It's hard to get a program before people realize the need for a program."

With an unbroken string of administrative successes behind him, Brown nevertheless gingerly approached his new assignment as vice president of the University of Chicago. Recognizing, with Montaigne, that only the fool is certain and assured, he had serious doubts about taking the job.

Money was no incentive. "I love a buck as much as anyone," Brown says, a trifle defensively, but the facts dispute this. Brown lives comfortably, but modestly, well within his salary. He buys clothes off the rack, drives a used car, and has absolutely no inclination toward yachts, stables or grand estates. It is a poorly kept secret that Brown has been offered–and has declined—positions in the health and prepayment field paying two and, on one specific occasion, three times as much as his present salary.

By remaining a hospital administrator and a teacher, Brown could easily have capped his career with distinction. Moving from hospital administration to university administration was risky. For one thing, there is inherent insecurity when one ventures into a new setting. Then, too, the great mass of factual knowledge Brown had accumulated in the health field would be of little use to him in making proper decisions outside this area.

On the other hand, the new position meant increased recognition to Brown and, ultimately, to all program trained hospital administrators.

Moreover, to turn down a challenging administrative position for personal reasons would have been, in effect, a repudiation of Brown's professional philosophy.

After weighing and assessing what he considered to be the

pertinent facts, Brown accepted the job and plunged into it wholeheartedly. As vice president, Brown is responsible, under University President George W. Beadle, for virtually all transactions involving the university that are not purely academic.

Now that his successors have been named, Brown has let go of his administrative assignments at the hospital and in the program of hospital administration, although he will continue his teaching assignments.

Brown also plans to remain close to national hospital affairs. "All university officials have some special identification," he explains, "and President Beadle expects me to retain my interest in the health field."

As Brown embarks on his new career as a top university official, he is discreetly mute about his future. Off his record, however, it seems unlikely that he has reached his professional peak.

What seems more likely is that somewhere in the Southeastern part of the country, which Brown loves and has never forgotten, lies a great university that will be looking for a new president in the next two or three or four years. When the name and performance of Ray Brown are brought forward, as they must be, chances are the university will study the facts, and stop looking.

And that, in the best Ray Brown tradition, is putting it impersonally.

Chapter Five

Ray E. Brown: The Early Chicago Years

Richard L. Johnson

My introduction to Ray was in 1948, when I entered the Graduate Program in Hospital Administration at the University of Chicago, At that time, he was the Superintendent of the University of Chicago Hospitals and Clinics and Associate Director of the Graduate Program. Academically, he was an Associate Professor in the School of Business. Dr. Arthur C. Bachmeyer was the Director of the program and Associate Dean of the Division of Biological Sciences. The following year, Dr. Bachmeyer retired and Ray became the Director of the program. In 1950, I joined him as Assistant Superintendent and Associate Director of the program. Our association continued through 1955 and our close personal friendship continued until his death. We wrote one book together, *Hospitals Visualized* (1957). From this perspective, I have many fond memories of the most remarkable person I have ever known.

Having grown up in North Carolina, where his father was a Baptist preacher, Ray had moved around from place to place as a child. Though he came from a family of several children, I can never recall any of his brothers or sisters visiting his home for a week or a weekend. While I never believed he had an unhappy childhood, he never dwelt on his childhood or his family. My own conclusion was that he was so taken up with the events of the day and what was happening in the health field that he never had time to look back.

In 1943, when Ray had finished his graduate work at the University of Chicago and earned his M.B.A., he returned to North Carolina to become Superintendent of North Carolina Baptist Hospital in Winston-Salem, North Carolina. In accepting that position, Ray believed he was offered a salary below what he thought he should be paid. He pointed this out to the board of trustees and offered a compromise—he would accept the salary ($6,000 per year) the first year and at the end of that period, if he had more than met the board's expectations with regard to his performance, he had the right to name his own salary for the second year. This was the agreement. At the end of the first year, the board agreed he had more than met their expectations and he could set his own salary. He did and named $12,000 per year. At the end of the second year at Baptist Hospital, Ray was invited by Dr. Bachmeyer to become Superintendent at the University of Chicago Hospitals and Clinics and moved to Chicago, only to encounter an unexpected problem.

Ray was on the job less than a week when Dr. Bachmeyer told him that Dr. Otis Whitecotton, his predecessor, had telephoned him and presented a dilemma. Dr. Whitecotton had resigned at the university to move to Ann Arbor as chief executive of the University of Michigan Hospitals. When he arrived, he discovered to his amazement that the position had two persons to fill it. There had been two separate groups, each of which thought it had the responsibility for filling the position. Both groups had carried out their assignments, and the two new superintendents arrived on the scene on the same day. At that point, Dr. Whitecotton placed a call to Dr. Bachmeyer, who told him to come on back to Chicago. He did and resumed the title of Superintendent, and Ray became the Assistant Superintendent while Dr. Whitecotton sought to get relocated. Within a short time, he moved to a position as chief executive of Highland-Alameda Hospital in Oakland, California, and Ray took over as Superintendent.

Ray was a workaholic. His work day started around 9 A.M. after a brisk walk from his apartment on Blackstone Avenue, a distance of about a mile. Always hatless, even in subzero weather, he would come into our office full of energy, ready to meet the day's challenges.

The day was filled with a stream of people, about half of whom were department heads, a mixture of senior and junior physicians wanting to discuss problems that were on their minds, and two or three times a week, outsiders from various health organizations seeking advice or assistance. In between visitors, Ray was constantly on the telephone calling and receiving calls from all across the United States—something that was done rarely in the early 1950s.

At 5 P.M. the outside office door was shut, and one of our two secretaries started taking dictation, which usually lasted until 7 o'clock, when we quit work for the day. This pattern was followed daily from Monday through Friday. Saturday was a scheduled half-day of work, which meant we usually left the hospital between 4 and 5 P.M. However, Saturdays were days when we had a good time at the hospital. At around 11 A.M., several of us would gather in Ray's office. The group usually included Irv Wilmot, Jim Connelly, and later, Dick Wittrup. Ray would analyze the events of the time that affected the health field, and put them in a theoretical framework, but always with a pragmatic twist that was easily recognizable as a practical answer to what was needed.

Ray's door was always open to physicians, administrative staff, department heads, and students in the graduate program. Some of the most fascinating discussions took place after the outer door was closed at 5 P.M. on weekdays. A knock on Ray's private office door often admitted Bob Ebert (later Dean of the Harvard Medical School), or another of Ray's contemporaries who just wanted to chat. Ray's availability, friendliness, and unfailing courtesy were the keys to his rapport with such associates.

Early in his career, Ray had developed his work habits. From Monday through Saturday, he was committed to his job and his professional field. Sundays were the family days—for Mary and the three girls. Mary was the strong pillar in the family, keeping track of all the activities and leaving Ray free to deal with the rest of the world. Ray and Mary were equals in every sense of the word, something that was largely unappreciated by outsiders because of Ray's reputation. Mary was well known to Ray's colleagues and friends, but her contributions to Ray's success were largely unknown.

December was always a month I hated while working with Ray. It was budget time. We often worked until 10 or 11 P.M., pouring over every departmental activity. In December, the afternoons were devoted to detailed, careful analysis of departmental activities and reviewing every aspect with the department head. When the department head left the meeting we would go to the cafeteria, eat dinner, and return to the conference room for our own work on the budget. This went on day after day for the entire month. Usually I would steal away for two hours on one of these December days to go downtown and do my Christmas shopping. If I didn't finish it within those two hours, I was out of luck for that season because there was no more time available. By the end of December, Ray really knew what was going on, what was needed. Then he made the necessary decisions to bring the organization into balance.

Ray treated the responsibilities of his position more seriously than any other person I have ever known. He took pride in running a good ship and making sure it ran smoothly. His success as an outstanding executive was partially due to his relationship with his boss, Lowell Coggeshall, the Dean of the Division of Biological Sciences. Dr. Coggeshall had been a leading authority on tropical medicine, but, when he became Dean, he understood that he had to totally give up clinical medicine and devote his full time to his administrative activities. Having made his decision, he never hedged on it. As a result, he had a deep appreciation of Ray's abilities as an executive. He saw his own role as being a downfield blocker for Ray, providing him the greatest organizational room possible to exercise his immense talent. To the best of my knowledge, Ray never took advantage of this relationship. Ray and Cog were an unbeatable combination, the result of which was a synergism that was well known and appreciated by the senior officers of the university.

In dealing with key personnel in the hospital, Ray had a sympathetic ear and was not adverse to bending the rules of the university. If a manager turned out to be incompetent and had to be replaced, Ray always kept the manager in his job until he was successfully relocated. While giving the appearance of being the dynamic, always ready to make a decision type, when it came to key personnel Ray was a marshmallow inside. He put up with inadequate performance while working to get the person relocated, without setting time limits unless he had come to the conclusion that the person was not making a serious effort to relocate.

No one that I knew was ever afraid of Ray. They might be awestruck by his intellect and capacity for work, but no one was ever fearful that Ray would be unfair or treat him or her in a demeaning way. Everybody was equal to Ray, to be treated with respect.

Ray could be tough when the situation demanded it. This toughness was an expression of his intellect, rather than any emotion. If someone such as the University Comptroller invaded his turf, or some other party in the central University Administration tried to take advantage of his authority, he went to all ends to prevent it. When those of us on his staff saw the problem as a minor breeze, Ray treated it as a raging storm, making us wonder why he devoted so much time and energy to the issue. Later, we all came to realize that he knew if he didn't blow the whistle then and there he would find his authority compromised later on and would be unable to do his job. From his perspective, better to take the time and devote his attention to the issue now and not have to spend more time and energy later.

Ray had two idiosyncrasies: In his early career he never wore a watch and seldom carried keys. Why he never wore a watch I could never determine, he was always asking someone the time or looking for a clock on a wall. The only key Ray carried was the key to his office. Even though the entire hospital was on one system with a master key that opened all the hundreds of doors in the medical center, Ray carried the key only to his own office. If he wished to inspect various areas, he would call Marie Neher, the Executive Housekeeper, to accompany him, because she was in charge of the keys.

While Ray gave his time freely and generously to his professional field, he never did it at the expense of his job as head of the hospital. An event occurred that typifies his commitment. We had attended a meeting together in San Antonio, Texas, and were returning to Chicago. Because of ice and rain, we didn't land at Midway Airport until 3:30 A.M., which meant we got home around 4:40 A.M.. Being tired, I stayed in bed until close to noon, when I arrived at the hospital. Ray had been at work since 9 A.M., believing it was his responsibility to be there on time.

Shortly after this occurred, I decided that I would match Ray stride for stride in terms of work effort. At the time I was 29 years old and Ray was 41. I kept up the pace for six months before throwing in the towel and acknowledging that I couldn't stand his pace.

In watching Ray dissect a management problem, I often thought of the process as though he had a banana and held it up, looked at it from all sides, and then quickly peeled the skin to get down to the meat of the problem. This speed and accuracy of his decision making was awesome, even after one had watched the process hundreds of times.

One afternoon, probably in 1954, Ray and I and Everett Johnson were together in his office, talking about the activities of the American College of Hospital Administrators and what needed to be done to make it a more dynamic organization. As ideas were expressed and debated, we began to focus on the need for an annual meeting, separate and apart from the Convocation, which was held on Sunday immediately preceding the opening of the annual American Hospital Association meeting, which was held each summer. We concluded that such a meeting would provide greater visibility to College affiliates by separating it from the AHA affairs.

Having decided this was a worthwhile idea, the question of when it should be held and how it should be structured came up. Ray turned around to the windowsill behind him, where he stacked the latest trade journals, picked up a copy of *Hospitals* magazine, and turned to the page listing state and regional conventions. As we scanned the page, it was evident that these meetings clustered in the fall and spring months but there was a gap during the winter. We all quickly agreed that February would be an ideal time for a meeting.

We next discussed how the meeting might be structured and concluded that a schedule of breakfast meetings organized around specific topics, with attendance at each seminar limited to a reasonable number of attendees, would permit all to participate. The more we talked, the better we liked the idea. But the problem of finding a hotel that could handle fifty or more for breakfasts simultaneously meant that the meeting would have to be in a major hotel. The three of us were familiar with the Palmer House in Chicago and quickly agreed that it probably would be the hotel of choice, if the meeting were to be held in Chicago. We recognized that February was a nasty month in Chicago, but saw this location as having two advantages: Chicago was in the middle of the United States and was one of the most accessible cities to reach from all parts of the country. In addition, because of the weather, attendees would be likely to stay inside the hotel, which meant we regarded Chicago as desirable.

With this "Congress concept" well in mind and outlined on paper, we turned our attention to the need for a journal to be published by the College. Again, the three of us thought that every professional society should have a scholarly publication on at least a quarterly basis. Advertising, if permitted, should be limited to the back cover. The articles should be ones submitted by affiliates of the College and screened by an editorial board.

By the time the afternoon was over, we had drafted our ideas on paper and Ray wrote a cover letter to Dean Conley, the Executive Director of the College, asking him to put these two ideas on the agenda for the next meeting of his governing board, where they were duly approved.

One of the interesting incidents in Ray's life took place when he left the University of Chicago Hospitals and went across the street to Central Administration as the number two officer of the university. This took place over Ray's objections.

When Lawrence Kimpton was retiring as President of the University of Chicago, the board of trustees established a search committee to seek a successor. The committee ultimately arrived at two names: George Beadle, a Nobel Prize winner in genetics, and Ray Brown. The decision focused on the issue of whether the university president should be a talented executive or a shining star in academic circles who would attract first rate academic talent to the facility. After much discussion, a compromise was reached. The top slot would be offered to George Beadle, and as part of the same action, the number two slot would be offered to

Ray as Chief Administrative Officer of the university. With that decision reached, George Beadle was offered and accepted the presidency of the university, and a committee of trustees met with Ray and offered him the number two slot. Ray politely declined, telling them he was totally satisfied with his present position.

But when George Beadle arrived on campus, he was instructed by the board of trustees to inform Ray that the board had voted him into the Chief Administrative Office position. Dutifully, Beadle carried out the wishes of the board. When that conversation took place, Ray, being the pragmatist he was, knew that he no longer had a choice to make; it had been taken out of his hands, and he reluctantly moved into Central Administration.

His three years in Central Administration were three of the worst years of his career. Ray was unhappy in that position from the day he took it until the day he left. On one occasion when we were together, Ray remarked that his job consisted of being in charge of all the janitorial services provided on the campus. His unhappiness stemmed from two sources. He was cut off from daily contact with the medical and hospital field and was forced to deal with administrative problems that held no interest for him. In addition, the imbalance between income and expense for the university as a whole meant that he had to control expenses at a level that was totally inadequate but within the revenue that could be generated. This was a condition totally different from the hospital, where he annually adjusted prices so that revenues would cover expenses. The result was a nightmare of frustration. Ray stuck it out for four years and then left to join the faculty at Duke University. He was so scarred by his experience that he insisted on a contract with Duke University that excluded him from having to deal with university administrative problems.

Many individuals who knew Ray only casually or from a professional association thought him to be a complex person. This was not the case at all. At the core of his being Ray was a man with simple values who operated from a well-defined set of personal principles. Ray believed that since he was honest and had integrity those with whom he dealt had the same sense of values. They had to prove to Ray that they didn't have them before he thought differently. Ray was not impressed with wealth or position as indicators of judgment. He made up his mind about those with whom he dealt based on his own observations.

Ray was fascinated with the management process and administrative behavior. For years, prior to writing his book, *Judgment in Administration* (1966), he was making notes, pondering the implications of good and bad administrative behavior, all the while wondering how to improve executive performance. The book, when finally published, was a distillation of ideas and thoughts that Ray had personally experienced and re-experienced, again and again. The hospital where he worked was his administrative laboratory. From every administrative encounter he found something to be learned. In a real sense, the book *Judgment in Administration* was a distillation of what Ray had learned over a quarter of a century as an executive.

The book never received the widespread recognition that was its due, probably because it was written by a hospital executive rather than a corporation executive. Yet, to my way of thinking, it ranks with *The Functions of the Executive*, published in 1938 and written about the management process.

The relationship of administrative and organizational theory to actual practice was clear to Ray. He would always challenge anyone who was foolish enough to say within earshot that something was fine in theory but not in practice. Ray would immediately remind the person that theory was only as good as it was in practice. A theory to be successful had to be workable over and over again in practice, or else the theory was not good theory. This was one of his favorite themes.

Ray's idea of how to relax was simply to get away to where he could think and put some kind of logic to the events in which he was participating. Ray was not a scholar in the classical sense. He firmly believed that hospital administration was, to put it in his words, "a practice." He saw no basic truths being derived from the field, which he believed was dependent on a number of disciplines that provided its foundation. He saw hospital administration drawing from organizational theory, economics, psychology, finance, sociology, theology, and medicine, among others. As a result of this, his 150 articles and two books were largely a collection of his insights developed out of his everyday work experiences. A review of his articles and books reveals very few footnotes and bibliographical references. Essentially, he reflected on what was happening and drew out of these experiences the elements that constituted sound administrative behavior and judgments.

Ray's influence is still being felt by those of us who knew him. Frequently, when experiencing a unique situation or in the middle of a hot discussion, the thought flashes through my mind, "I sure wish Ray was here so I could talk this over with him."

Ray had little interest in hobbies or avocations. He considered golf his main sport and probably averaged no more than four or five rounds every summer. When on the course he pursued a golf ball as though it were a management problem to be quickly solved. He played rapidly, with the same degree of energy and vigor he exhibited in the office, making quips about the game as he toured the course.

To the best of my knowledge, Ray never followed an exercise program, but his weight never varied because he watched what he ate, and never overate. He smoked throughout his entire adult life, and there was always a pack of Camel cigarettes sitting on his desk.* The only time he stopped smoking was when he was hospitalized for a heart condition. This didn't last long, and shortly after leaving the hospital he went back to smoking again. He did this with full knowledge of the medical implications, but decided he was going to go on living the same vigorous, energetic life he had always led, doing the things he had always done, right up to the point where it finally caught up with him. This was a deliberate, rational judgment on his part. Ray was 61 years of age when he died. George Bugbee summed it up succinctly and accurately when he said, on learning of Ray's death, "This country has just lost a national resource."

References

Chester I. Barnard, *The Functions of the Executive* (Cambridge, MA: Harvard University, 1938).

*Later, Ray switched to Winstons, another R. J. Reynolds Tobacco Company product.

Ray E. Brown, *Judgment in Administration* (New York: McGraw-Hill, Inc., 1966; Second Edition: Pluribus Press, Division of Teach'em, Inc., and American College of Hospital Administrators, 1982).

Ray E. Brown and Richard Johnson, *Hospitals Visualized: A Text for Use with Field Trips in Teaching Hospital Administration,* 2d ed. (Chicago: American College of Hospital Administrators, 1957).

Chapter Six

Ray E. Brown: The Duke Years, 1964–1974

Donald S. Smith

Ray came to Duke in 1964 and started an association that lasted the rest of his life. He was scheduled to arrive on July 1, and the suite of offices that was to house the Program in Hospital Administration, as it was then known, was not scheduled for completion until around that date. As the time for his arrival got closer, it kept getting earlier, and he ultimately arrived in early April. Possibly this reflected his dissatisfaction with his job at the University of Chicago and a desire to get on to other things. It may also have been a happy anticipation of a return to North Carolina, where he had grown up, gone to college, and begun his career in hospital administration, or perhaps just the rising to a new challenge.

My first meeting with Ray was an eye-opener. Casually I asked him where he was living, and he said, "1207 Woodburn." I asked him what kind of house it was and he said that he did not know, adding, "Mary bought it. She always buys our houses. I'll see it when our furniture arrives." His statement that he moved into a lot of houses he had never seen is, to me, entirely plausible.

Because his office was not ready, Ray was given a desk, chair, file cabinet, and telephone in what is now the lobby of the Diagnostic and Treatment Building, then nearing completion. It was across the street from Duke Hospital, and Ray was the only one in the building who was not a construction worker. The lobby was finished, so Ray did not have to dodge painters, but he probably had the largest office at Duke University. It really did not matter, as Ray seldom had visitors when he was there, which was not often in the early days. He had committed to a heroic speaking schedule before leaving Chicago, and he was away much of the time.

The program that Ray had become director of had been in existence for less than two years, and had not graduated a class, and was not yet accredited. I was to be the only other full-time faculty member, although not officially until July 1. There were some eight graduates of the predecessor program, a nondegree, certificate program, but there was no alumni organization for the certificate-holders. Ray had no secretary, only part-time assistance from the hospital director's office. There was no departmental classroom or library.

This is not to say that Duke was remiss in its preparations. Departmental space was under construction, and a secretarial position was budgeted, but all the planning was based on a July 1 timetable, and Ray was off and running ahead of that schedule. Of course the authorities at Duke had agreed to Ray's early arrival and knew he was coming, but the immutability of the construction schedule gave the early days a rather *ad hoc* aura.

Ray was not impeded by the lack of departmental facilities. He immediately got onto the teaching schedule, conducting a first-year weekly seminar on management, and a second-year seminar on trends in the health care field. He plunged into the preparations for an accreditation visit. And he joined in the selection of an incoming class, which led to my first and only confrontation with Ray.

Duke had set a target of twelve students per class, and we had offered admission to twelve at a point in time, although we had not received commitments to enroll from all twelve. An additional applicant appeared on campus through a misunderstanding, so we assembled the Admissions Committee and interviewed the unexpected applicant—in Ray's absence, as we had been instructed to do. We were very impressed with the applicant, and voted to admit him, even though it might mean a class of thirteen, as it ultimately did.

When Ray heard about this decision made in his absence, he gave me the most thorough verbal shredding that I have ever received. I had been instructed to make decisions in his absence, and thought I had been doing what was expected of me, but apparently he did not see it that way. Later what Ray seemed to be saying was that he—and he alone—was going to run the Program. Much later I came to think he was becoming aware at that time that Duke was not going to turn out as he had expected, and was beginning to develop frustrations. Probably it was bad timing, and Ray did not ask if I had tried to reach him about the decision; I had. I think he felt it was a case of pre-Brown Duke letting him down.

The case was closed. Ray never brought it up again, and we never had heated differences again. It is ironic, I think, that the thirteenth student is one of the three Duke alumni editors of the Brown papers that appear earlier in this publication, and is one of the "Dukies" for whom Ray ultimately developed the highest esteem.

During this time, Ray learned of a project under development by the Hospital Research and Educational Trust (HRET), the not-for-profit foundation of the American Hospital Association. The W. K. Kellogg Foundation would give HRET money to make grants to five Centers of Hospital Continuing Education, these to be established by educational centers to conduct continuing education for hospital personnel in specific geographical areas. Ray developed a proposal for such a center at Duke, aimed at teaching management to hospital executives in the Carolinas–Virginias area.

The proposal brought together a number of features that made a lot of sense. Ray had already committed to doing an annual management seminar for the Tennessee Hospital Association that fall, so we had a chance at a "dry run." The Carolinas–Virginias Hospital Conference was still in existence, so we had a congruent administrative structure with which to deal. Ray's reputation was, of course, a major factor. The proposal was accepted.

One of our early steps in implementing the Center was to attend a meeting of the Carolina-Virginia Executive Committee to obtain their support and outline the Center's potential. The meeting was set at the Greenbriar at White Sulphur Springs, W.V., in early June of 1964. It turned out that the meeting was the day following the scheduled accreditation visit by the Association of University Programs in Hospital Administration (AUPHA). We completed the accreditation visit about 5:00 P.M., then jumped into Ray's car and headed for White Sulphur Springs, full of elation because we had been assured that we would be accredited. (Things were much simpler then.)

We ate dinner at a restaurant south of Roanoke, Va. It was getting late, and we were getting tired. We studied the map and noticed a road that ran directly from Roanoke to White Sulphur Springs. Ordinarily we would have continued north to Clifton Forge, Va., then headed west to White Sulphur Springs, but the alternative route represented the hypotenuse of the triangle. Always ready for something simpler, Ray said, "Let's try it." We did, with me at the wheel.

The road we followed was Virginia Route 311, and all take note: It is one of the twistiest, narrowest, most precipitous roads in the Southeast, possibly in the nation. Worse, it got foggy. We dragged into the Greenbriar at about 1:00 A.M. Our joint attitude was churlish, and it was not improved by finding that there was only one twin bedded room left. Ray and I had traveled together a lot already, and both knew that we preferred single rooms; Ray explained that he liked to read and write late, and I was quite candid in enjoying television. But it was, as Ray said, "Any old port in a storm," and probably too late for him to want to read anyway, so we took the room together.

Ray may have preferred to read and write, but he was a prodigious snorer. He slept soundly, and noisily, the entire night, while I lay quietly awake. We attended the morning meeting of Carolinas–Virginias, and headed back to Durham with me still at the wheel. As we passed the intersection with Va. 311, heading for Clifton Forge, Ray said, "Whose idea was it to take that road?" The question was rhetorical.

Ray was interested in cars. The one he bought when he moved to Durham—I do not know if he owned a car in Chicago—

was a sporty Chevy II with bucket seats, a console, and a big engine. He enjoyed driving, and driving fast. The reason that I drove most of the time when we travelled by car was that Ray had had occasional brushes with the law, and was always leery of accumulating more violations points. When he did drive, he drove extremely well—and fast.

The only time I heard him mention any family other than wife Mary and his daughters was one time when we were driving back from a meeting. Possibly reflecting on his driving record, he abruptly said, "My brother-in-law owns a go-cart race track in Raleigh. We ought to go. We can drive as fast as we want and not get a ticket."

In June of 1964, the departmental offices were completed, and we moved into the second floor of Baker House, one of the Medical Center buildings attached to Duke Hospital. Ray and I each had an office, and there was a secretarial office between us, with a pass-through window into each of our faculty offices. We also had a large conference room and library near the main suite.

We hired our first full-time secretary, Linda Pethia, the wife of a junior Duke faculty member. (Linda was later to graduate from college and join Ray in Phi Beta Kappa, something I believe would have pleased him greatly.) Linda was the only secretary that Ray had while at Duke, and he considered her outstanding.

By this time, Ray had largely completed the speaking engagements he had accepted while still at Chicago, and was in Durham most of the time. He began regularly to join the Duke Hospital administrative staff for lunch. The group typically included Charlie Frenzel, Administrative Director of Duke Hospital (and eventually Ray's successor as Program Director); Charlie Boone, Assistant Administrative Director; Ralph Jennings, also Assistant Administrative Director; and Jim Anderson, Chief Fiscal Officer.

Ray enjoyed a good argument; he was aggressive, well informed, and a great needler. His favorite fellow debater was Charlie Boone, and Jim Anderson could occasionally be drawn in. The others usually were content to listen. The topic did not matter, and Ray and Charlie took opposite sides. The debates were heated; the voices would get high and the faces red. Neither would admit that the other was right. Yet they were the best of friends and remained so after both had left Duke.

Ray was interested in sports, and followed local athletics closely. Although he had attended arch-rival North Carolina, he took a great interest in Duke athletics. When Ray and Charlie Boone were not arguing, the discussion often was about Duke athletics. For some reason, Ray never baited Charlie Boone about North Carolina's athletic successes against Duke, although Charlie had graduated from Duke and lived and died with its teams. Perhaps Ray felt that this would be taken too personally.

Ray was always looking for sports analogies to apply to management, although I never heard him use one. One day we talked about Gene Bearden, who won twenty games for the Cleveland Indians in 1948 to help win the pennant. His strike-out pitch was a knuckle ball which was virtually unhittable but also was almost out of the strike zone. This was picked up late in the 1948 season, and by 1949 the word had gotten around to lay off Bearden's knuckler. He was soon gone from the majors. Ray was intrigued, and said he was sure he could use that example. Long afterward he said that he could never figure out how to use it.

In the fall of 1964, Ray began to develop the National Forum on Hospital and Health Affairs. He envisioned a meeting of national health leaders to discuss a single topic, not to attempt to develop a solution, but rather to try to define issues and assess the state of the relevant practice. That Forum would be held on the Duke campus, in a University classroom, and it would be strictly an invitational meeting—and no alternates accepted.

Ray submitted a proposal to the Duke Endowment to sponsor the Forum, and the Endowment accepted. The main part of the Endowment sponsorship was to publish and distribute printed proceedings, and the Endowment still supports this undertaking.

Ray told me that when he was selecting the dates for the first Congress on Administration, he picked the winter weekend when the Chicago weather was most often the worst. He said he wanted terrible weather so people would want to stay indoors and, hopefully, discuss administration. He told me to find out which weekend in May in Durham weather had the best chance of being nice. He wanted the word to get out how beautiful North Carolina was that time of year so a lot of people would want to come.

The first Forum was set on the second weekend of May 1965 and was hailed as very much of a success. There were seventy-odd participants, mostly personal friends of Ray's and an excellent representation of the leadership of the health field of the middle sixties. And the weather was perfect.

While the Forum was under development, Ray was very much on the go. He continued a heavy speaking calendar, scheduling all his classes on Thursday and Friday so he was free to commit for the first three days of the week. He was scrupulous about meeting class. He often was something of a shock to the students—they sometimes found his pragmatic style a bit much to swallow. They initially thought him to be cynical and pessimistic, cold and unsympathetic. By the time they were ready to graduate, however, their attitudes toward him approached adulation. It was a rare student who was not won over to his outlook.

At the same time, the Center of Hospital Continuing Education was getting going. The first presentation was made in Durham at the now-defunct Washington Duke Hotel, and dealt with computer applications for administrators. It was conducted by the Department of Industrial Engineering of the University of Michigan, and was a lead-in to programs for hospital department heads on an industrial engineering-based staffing methodology for hospital departments. These meetings were held in Roanoke, Va., for the Virginia and West Virginia hospitals, and in Charlotte, N.C., for North and South Carolina. This series continued for three years.

Ray was also engaged in the setting up of management seminars for Carolinas–Virginias hospitals. North Carolina and South Carolina chose to combine for a joint management seminar to be held on the Duke campus, while West Virginia had its own at the Greenbriar. There Ray and I had separate rooms. The approach was to take a single element of management—delegation, span of control, and so on—and develop a two-and-a-half-day meeting around this theme. The following year a second topic would be similarly developed. The faculty was Ray and me plus such other faculty members from Duke as could make contributions.

In addition to the Carolinas-Virginias seminars, series were conducted by the state hospital associations of Louisiana, Tennessee, Oklahoma, and Mississippi. On top of this, Ray arranged for management development programs at Veterans Administration hospitals at Durham, Fayetteville, Oteen, and Salisbury, North Carolina, and at Dublin, Georgia.

While I was then Coordinator of the Center for Hospital Continuing Education on paper, Ray really was the Center. He made the contacts, set the dates, developed the curriculum, and was the star speaker. He was a great drawing-card, and no seminar in which he was featured was ever cancelled or rescheduled for lack of response. While I did a lot of legwork and spent a great deal of time travelling—I once had to look out the window of my motel to figure out where I had awakened—it was Ray who made the thing work.

Other than the teaching programs, Ray did not seem very interested in making things go at Duke. For him it was a time to think, to write, and to teach. He finished *Judgment in Administration* while at Duke, and had it published in 1966, and completed portions of two other books. He enjoyed his interactions with the Duke Hospital administrative staff, most of whom held part-time faculty status and taught details about running hospitals while Ray dealt with management theory and major issues of the health field. In fact, his title at Duke was Professor of Administration, not Hospital Administration. And he enjoyed every opportunity to teach, especially the Duke graduate students.

There was not a lot to the management of the M.H.A. program, and Ray was content to leave most of that to me. I have always had a feeling that Ray came to Duke with the expectation that the Program was going to be more than it was to become, and that something happened. He may have been unduly optimistic, promises may have been made that could not be delivered, or there may have been misunderstandings. I never did find out. Perhaps he was still so disenchanted with university administration by his Chicago experience that he temporarily avoided it.

And if he was less than entirely happy at Duke, he never let it show. He was, after all, a Southerner, and back in the South, where b-u-s-i-n-e-s-s is pronounced "bidness" and people knew where I was from when Ray said I was from VERmont. (I am from New Hampshire. Ray knew that and he knew it annoyed me when he said VERmont. But he always said it with a twinkle in his eye. He was quite a tease.)

Once I asked Ray why he left University of Chicago administration, and he said it was because it was dull compared to hospitals and he needed some time to think and write. I asked him if the next step would be to run a university and he said, "I thought so until I was able to watch the president of the University of Chicago from up close. Most of the job was asking people for money, and I'm not interested in spending my time doing that."

On another occasion I asked him if he wanted to be a consultant, and he said, "Never. Consultants are people who spend their nights in motel rooms writing up what they spend the day talking about. That's not for me." Yet he was always willing to hear people out on their proposals and give advice. He was frequently consulted by top administration at the Duke University Medical Center, and once he hosted a group of state hospital association executives to consult on the future directions of these organizations.

Prior to 1967, the Association of University Programs in Hospital Administration (AUPHA) held its annual meeting on University campuses, with the programs taking turns as hosts. At the 1965 meeting at Cornell, Ray was asked to serve as president for 1965–1966. He talked to me before accepting, asking if we could handle the hosting of the 1966 annual meeting. Flattered by his consideration, I assured him we could.

Ray agreed to serve, and was named the AUPHA President. AUPHA was a small organization of probably 14 to 16 program directors at that time, occasionally somewhat derisively referred to as the "Director's Club." Despite its small size, it was considered a very prestigious group because of its exclusivity, rightly or wrongly. In any case, Ray seemed to take it pretty much in stride, although apparently he was very flattered. What was striking about it is that it made him one of those extremely rare individuals who had served as the elected head of the American College of Hospital Administrators, the American Hospital Association, and the Association of University Programs in Hospital Administration.

The 1966 AUPHA annual meeting was held on the Duke campus. It was the last of the on-campus meetings. At the meeting, AUPHA, apparently at least partially at Ray's behest, decided to end the on-campus meetings and meet as other national organizations did, ending the "Director's Club" image. The meeting also marked the introduction of Gary Filerman as the Executive Director of AUPHA. Furthermore, the meeting honored the retirement of James A. Hamilton, the long-time Director of the Minnesota program. Ray presided over these sessions, with considerable aplomb, and did not seem to mind sharing the stage with Jim Hamilton.

The 1966 Forum was held in May, and drew a larger audience than the first one. The first Forum had dealt with the topic "Multiple Hospital Units Under Single Management." The topic of the second was "The Hospital Patient Outside the Hospital," and examined such areas as home care, extended care facilities, and other alternatives to inpatient care managed by inpatient care facilities. The topic of the program in each case was selected and organized by Ray. Ray has been described as being 20 years ahead of his time; might these not have been topics of the middle 1980s?

1966 saw the introduction of Medicare, and one of the Center's programs was what was expected to be a modest session on the implementation of Medicare, featuring Ray, a speaker from HEW, a third party representative, and a hospital representative. The meeting, which was expected to draw about 40, had a turnout of about 200. One point came out of the meeting: as just about everyone answered each question differently, there still was a lot to learn.

Ray and Medicare were linked. In 1965 a call came in to the office. I was talking to Linda in the central office when the phone rang. She said, "Hello." There was a pause, and she asked, "Of what?" There was another brief pause and she said "Oh." She buzzed Ray's line, and he opened the pass-through window and asked who was calling. Linda said, "The President is calling." Ray said, "The president of what?" She said, "The President of the United States." Ray said, "Oh."

President Lyndon Johnson was calling to ask Ray to come to talk with him personally about the proposed Medicare legislation. Ray was one of several health field leaders who went to talk with President Johnson and who were asked in one by one to speak directly with the President. Ray supported Medicare, explaining that health insurance was like term insurance from a job, and that when you retired, it ended. When he got back his only comment about the President was, "He was very cordial, and he's a lot bigger and more powerful-looking than he seems to be on television." The President later sent Ray one of the pens he had used to sign Medicare legislation. Ray's initial reaction was an impish grin as he wrote with the pen to see if there was still ink in it.

The graduate students loved Ray, at least once they recovered from his initial impact. He was always available when in town, and he would talk with an unexpected caller right up to his next appointment. Always friendly and sympathetic, he was also brutally candid, and they appreciated it. Probably the phrase he used most with them was, "Life is real and life is earnest."

Ray tended to speak in, if not in cliches, at least time-worn phrases. He knew he was doing it, and did not apologize. Rather he defended his words, saying the reason that they had been around so long was that they made sense and were true. There was a lot of pragmatism to him. Once a visitor left a raincoat, and Ray went to great lengths to find the owner. He noticed that the label was from a New Haven store, so he reviewed his calendar and called everyone who had visited in the past six months who was from anywhere near New Haven, but without finding the owner. Finally he said, "Don, there's only one thing to do about this coat—see which one of us it fits best." Thus I acquired a fine raincoat.

Ray was a smoker as along as I knew him, and when he was at Duke he smoked Winstons. At a very gourmet banquet given by the Toronto program at the 1964 AUPHA meeting, diners were requested not to smoke during the meals as it would ruin their palates and insult the chef, and so no ashtrays would be provided. After just about every course, and there were many, Ray would make his excuses and to go the men's room, which was directly off the banquet room. He would be gone a few minutes. When he came out, billows of smoke would follow him out the door. He would just shrug his shoulders and give us that impish grin.

He always lit his cigarettes with book matches. I asked him why he did not get a lighter. He said, "I've got a drawer full of them. People keep giving them to me." When I asked him why he did not use one, he said, "I can look at a book of matches and know how many lights I have left. I can't do that with a lighter." That struck me as pragmatic.

Ray seemed to be always thinking and always writing. His notes on any topic frightened me. His habit was to have a file for a topic, and when he had a thought, he would write it on whatever was available, put it in his pocket, and take it home and file it. His files were filled with just about every imaginable sort of paper—expended match books, paper napkins, scratch pad leaves from seemingly hundreds of hotels and motels. His handwriting was, as he said, "sort of ugly but easy to read." None of us ever had any trouble understanding his scribbles.

Later in his career, Ray always wore a watch. He wore it on the back of his left wrist parallel to the back of his hand and, as he always wore long-sleeved shirts, he had a characteristic way of bending his left wrist down while pushing up his left sleeve with his right hand. The watch was always the same one, a simple gold one with hands and a leather strap. He always wore a two-piece business suit, a white shirt with button cuffs, and a conservative tie. While I knew Ray for 10 years, I cannot recall him wearing anything else, anywhere. And I never saw him wear a hat.

Ray's dealings with people were at all times courteous and courtly, reflecting, I believe, that he was really a humble person. He could get pretty forceful in a debate and had a derisive snort that he used to good advantage, but he never got personal. He seldom used coarse language; once in a while he said "damn" or "hell," although never while lecturing to a group. He observed good etiquette and expected it from others. If he did not get it, he was annoyed—the surest way to be dropped from the Forum invitation list, in perpetuity, was to fail to respond to his invitation.

In addition to bad manners, things that really annoyed him were sloppy thinking and sentimentality. He was an unusually clear and precise thinker, and I never heard anything sentimental from him. Perhaps he considered sentiment antithetic to pragmatism, and he was proud of his pragmatism. "A lot of damn foolishness," was his evaluation of poor thinking or sentimentality.

Ray had a way of being courtly and "country" at the same time. He knew the Southern idiom, and would talk it for hours. Yet, in the turbulent 1960s, he would not tell ethnic jokes, nor speak unkindly of any particular group that was making headlines in those days. Individuals in those days of heated rhetoric were not exempt from his scorn, no matter what their allegiance. The more illogical or absurd the allegation, the greater his derision. And he was not patient with defenders of the status quo; he knew change when he saw it. Truly unsentimental, he did not appear to resent change but seemed most interested in adjusting to it. When a well-qualified woman applicant for the Program, Mary M. Blanks, appeared in the spring of 1966, Ray insisted that she be considered like anyone else, although Duke had not had a woman graduate student in this field before. She was subsequently admitted with Ray's strong backing. Routine now, but rather heady for the 1960s.

The pace continued the following year. The Center was going strong, Ray was still speaking all over the place, the Thursday–Friday class schedule was still observed, the 1967 Forum ("Capital Financing of Hospitals—Sources and Concerns") was a great success, we were starting to get requests for earlier Forum proceedings as they began to appear in bibliographies, enrollment in the M.H.A. program had grown from the nine in the first class to fourteen, Ray had organized the alumni to the point that they had regular meetings, elected officers, and a governing authority—and had chosen Ray as the first official Honorary Member.

Then Ray announced that he was leaving Duke in the fall to assume the chief executive position at the Harvard-affiliated hospitals. The shock was there, but no one was overwhelmed. It had seemed too good to be true, and we had all felt it could not last. Ray explained his decision by saying, "When I came to Duke, I was ready to settle down to teaching and writing. Now I miss having a big organization to push around. I want the excitement of running a hospital, and I doubt that I'll get this big a challenge again."

Charlie Frenzel, Administrative Director of Duke Hospital and Professor of Hospital Administration, was chosen as Ray's successor, to assume office in several months as he phased out of running the hospital. Charlie was a good choice and had a favorable impact on the program during the next three years before he, too, started missing the big organization to push around and returned to running hospitals.

Before he left, Ray sat down with Charlie and proposed that he, Ray, continue to run the Forum. Ray would plan the program, select and invite the speakers, and edit the proceedings. The Program would provide the meeting and housing arrangements, make the mailings, and arrange the printing of the proceedings. The offer was accepted. Ray and Charlie were good friends, and the arrangement was comfortable. The 1968, 1969, and 1970 Forums went on as usual. Ray was very much in evidence at the Forums, and I suspect that if an individual came to Duke only for the Forum, everything would have looked the same.

Late in 1971, Charlie Frenzel resigned to accept the chief executive position at a multi-unit system in the Philadelphia area. Among the early decisions made on Charlie's resignation was that Ray would continue to develop and run the Forum, at least for 1972 and until the future direction of the Program was clarified. I was left in the position of Program Director *pro tem*, and the only full-time faculty member. Among my early phone calls was one from Ray Brown. I told Ray that I felt as though I had been made the captain of the Titanic about 100 feet from the iceberg, and his reply was, "Don't worry, Don. I've faced some pretty terrible things in my life. And most of them didn't even happen."

In the spring of 1972, B. Jon Jaeger, a 1964 graduate of the M.H.A. program who had subsequently earned a Ph.D. at Duke, was named to head the Program; the Program was named a department of the Medical Center, and Jon became the Chairman. I was very pleased at the selection, as I knew and respected Jon. I was also very pleased at one of Jon's early moves—getting Ray to agree to continue to mastermind the Forum, and also getting Ray to agree to serve as a regular visiting faculty member.

Under this new arrangement, Ray would not only carry on with the Forum, but he would spend a day each week in classes with second-year students, conducting a seminar on management. It was almost like 1964–1967 again. Ray seemed very enthusiastic about the arrangement. He was faithful to his agreement, invariably appearing at Duke on schedule, whatever the weather or demands on his time, initially to traumatize, then proselytize, graduate students. The Forums continued, generally hailed as farseeing and timely. Some of the attendees had been to the first Forum and had almost never missed one—Cleve Rodgers and Dave Kinzer come to mind, and there probably are others.

When Ray was in town, I made a point of seeing him as much as possible. He always asked me how things were in "VERmont." He was often over for dinner, and was good for some conversation before early retirement "to read and think." He did not say much about Harvard except to say that it had not taken him long to figure out that he was not going to be able to work that one out and, in his opinion, "the person who can hasn't been born yet."

Ray was at my house for dinner the last night he spent in Durham, that being in late April, 1974, after he had returned to Chicago to head the McGaw Medical Center at Northwestern University. He thought the beef short ribs were excellent, but claimed the horseradish sauce would give him an ulcer and he would have to quit after three servings. Northwestern-McGaw was going fine, he thought, and he would soon get things running right. We reviewed Duke athletics, probably agreeing to wait until next year. Ray mentioned that he had a new hobby, collecting antique brass. After asking my permission, he turned over every piece of brass in the room to read the symbols on the bottom. The next day I drove him to the airport, and left him saying, "I'll see you at the Forum." The tenth Forum was about three weeks away.

When Ray died on May 4, I was in New Hampshire on the way back from an accreditation visit to Cornell, and did not hear about it until I returned to Durham. I later learned that he and Mary had been on a brass-hunting trip to a flea market, and that he had died during a nap after they got home. Because of my late return from the Cornell trip, I did not attend Ray's funeral in Chicago, but Jon Jaeger did, and he and I drove to Cherryville, N.C., for the interment services a few days later.

During the ride to Cherryville, Jon said, "Ray and I were discussing his returning to Duke when he got Northwestern-McGaw running smoothly. I really believe he would have come." After a long and thoughtful pause he said, "Well, so much for that idea now."

Ray's remains were buried in the churchyard of a church that Ray's father had once served. A number of the long-time Duke people were there—Charlie Boone was there, and Zach Thomas, who published a classic description of the service.

The headstone was small and elegantly simple. It was about twelve inches wide and six inches high, designed to fit flush with the earth, and read "Ray Everette Brown, September 16, 1913–May 4, 1974." Mary pointed out that the middle name was misspelled—Everett was correct—and that she would have to get it redone. I think Ray would have gotten it right the first time.

Immediately after Ray's death, the Duke University Department of Health Administration assembled funds, some from university sources, some from the alumni, some from other friends, to create the Ray E. Brown Scholarship. While the principal is still growing, the scholarship has annually granted a modest award to a deserving graduate student in health administration.

The 1974 National Forum, which had been put together by Ray as all the previous Forums were, was conducted as scheduled. Some consideration was given to postponing it because it fell only a few days after his death, but the consensus was that Ray was a very pragmatic person and would have insisted that it go on. Other than a brief eulogy and a moment of silence, and the announcement of the Ray E. Brown Scholarship, the format was essentially unchanged then and in the 13 subsequent Forums.

The same year, the Duke University Hospital and Health Administration Alumni Association (DUHHAAA) established the Ray E. Brown Memorial Lecture. Presented annually at the DUHHAAA meeting on the Duke University campus in the fall, the lectureship has featured a number of old friends of Ray's, including Dick Wittrup, Irv Wilmot, Bob Cunningham, Charlie Boone, Mary Blanks, Ev Johnson, and Alex McMahon. The lecture has served partly as a eulogy to Ray, and partly to present an important speaker on a current health or management topic.

Mary Brown, Ray's widow, subsequently moved back to Durham, N.C., and still resides there. She is invited annually to attend the Ray E. Brown Memorial Lecture, as is daughter Norvell Brown Kennedy, who with her husband runs a business in Durham. Mary and Norvell have been guests of the Alumni Association at a number of presentations.

CHAPTER SEVEN

THE BOSTON PERSPECTIVE

Richard Wittrup

Ray Brown spoke the language of management and made his reputation in that field. But his personality and style were, in my view, those of a 1950s-style Southern politician. He had the urge for recognition, the respect for power, and the sense of social structure inherent in that culture. Given the right opportunity, he might have been the United States Senator from North Carolina, a role he could have performed with considerable distinction.

Pattern of Delegation

One of Ray's great contributions was his perception of the hospital as a product of the social forces that shaped it. Consistent with that view, his management efforts gave priority to the maintenance of relationships with the medical staff and his administrative superiors in the university.

The rest of his time was spent on his academic interests and responsibilities, the American Hospital Association, the American College of Hospital Administrators, and other outside activities.

He paid attention to internal operations to the extent that they affected medical staff, university, or other relationships.

Beyond that, I think it is fair to say that he was not very interested. He made few contributions in the areas of hospital programs, management techniques, or organizational structure that I can recall.

Thus there is not much to be said about this approach to delegation insofar as he managed a hospital along traditional lines and expected people to do their work. When something caught his attention he did not hesitate to meddle, but he didn't have time to do it much.

When one of us was sent to deal with an outside party, Ray was careful to establish the "party line" in advance and got furious if it was departed from. We were not sent to negotiate or make decisions. I hated such assignments, because all I could do was sit there and repeat what I was told to say. If something new came up, I had to go back for instructions.

Pattern of Internal Communication

Ray held weekly department head meetings. As I recall, they were mostly gripe sessions and not very productive. My feeling at the time was that they bored him but were something he thought every administrator had to do.

Ray probably thought he was accessible, but the problem was that he never had any time. It often took days to get an appointment, and when you finally got into his office he spent three-fourths of the time of the telephone.

Ray was sensitive about what people said. Any remark that might be considered critical of him or might give others a basis for criticism drove him up the wall. If his people made such a remark, they could count on a royal chewing-out within an hour of his hearing about it.

Maintaining Accountability

Ray was big on budgets. He spent three or four weeks every year in budget development. For his administrative subordinates and department heads, it was an ordeal. Females often came out crying. Males felt like it.

But once the budget was set it was the Bible, and woe unto anyone who did not live within it. Asking for a mid-year increase was a definite no-no. He would check up on things that interested him but I don't recall that there was any particular pattern to it.

Consultation

Ray was a careful decision maker and, as I recall, did a lot of consulting when something important was cooking. He had no trouble making decisions, but he loved to argue, which he did aggressively and with great skill. This intimidated many of his subordinates, who too often capitulated, even when he was wrong. I found it stimulating. Appointments being so difficult to get, I fell into the pattern of stopping by his office after the secretaries had gone home for the day. When we got into a topic that interested him, we might stay until eight o'clock. Our wives didn't particularly appreciate it.

Response to Bad Decisions

On matters of significance, Ray didn't make bad decisions. The only ones that come to mind are his decision to join the University of Chicago Central Administration and his decision to go to Boston. He got out of both by leaving.

I do not recall any attempts to justify a bad decision or to find a face-saving way out. From what I know of Ray, he would have been the first to recognize a bad call, would have taken it seriously but in good humor, and then would have reversed field as quickly and as gracefully as possible.

Like most of his contemporaries in the emerging field of hospital administration, Ray started at the top and had no hands-on experience in the nuts and bolts of hospital operations. This did not inhibit his self-confidence in making decisions on detailed operating questions. Consequently, on such matters he was often wrong, but never in doubt. Fortunately, the hospitals he ran were big, and his bad instructions could be sterilized by his underlings before they caused any harm.

Approachability

I would not characterize Ray as being either gregarious or isolated. He was not the kind of administrator who walked around the hospital visiting with his staff. My first job at the University of Chicago was as a typist and, later, as supervisor of a stenographic pool that transcribed discharge summaries. It was just across the corridor from his office. I think I worked there a year before I knew who he was.

Ray was neither aloof nor arrogant, but he did not believe in cultivating personal relationships with his employees. Many were afraid of him. He was from the South. He thought it was the job of bosses to boss, of employees to obey, and of everyone to respect his place. The University of Chicago was unionized. He didn't like labor unions, never accepted their legitimacy, and never dealt with them directly if he could avoid it.

Patience with Poor Performers

Generally speaking, Ray did not surround himself with strong subordinates, and a number of them were uncommonly weak. One can count on the fingers of one hand the number of people who worked for him and later went on to make national reputations. With a few exceptions, his subordinates never did anything outstanding, and that seemed to be okay with him.

I was with him in Chicago for about four years. I remember one person being fired by him, and that was for doing something dishonest, not for performing poorly.

Ray as Teacher

Ray was a marvelous teacher, as his hospital administration students will attest. He was an equally good teacher to his administrative subordinates. However, he taught by the Socratic method, and the pupil had to hold up his end of the dialogue. Few of his subordinates had the ability to do that.

Pleasure and Grief

Ray quite obviously got his main enjoyment from the Graduate Program in Hospital Administration, writing, giving speeches, and participating in organizational affairs such as those of the American Hospital Association and the American College of Hospital Administrators. I don't recall anything in particular that gave him grief, unless it was when a graduate program alumnus got into trouble. He supported them all, winners and losers, and I expect he lost sleep over some of the latter. In other cases, he had the ability to avoid things he didn't like, or else to do something about them. If he agonized, he didn't show it.

Medical Staff

Ray viewed the medical staff as any successful politician would view a powerful constituency. He had their respect, but he knew his place. He accurately read and carefully cultivated the power structure, never interfered in their prerogatives, and never got into confrontations.

I remember that we had one famous doctor (he ultimately won a Nobel Prize) who did not believe in discharge summaries and would not let his residents do them. Ray looked the other way.

It has to be remembered that the University of Chicago had a very good medical school and that all members of the medical staff were full-time faculty members. Thus Ray did not have the kind of medical staff problems that were common in community hospitals at the time.

Ray had few close personal friends, but during the latter part of his life, the ones he had were his contemporaries from the University of Chicago medical school faculty.

Work Habits

Ray was a classic workaholic. His work was his life. He got up in the morning and went to the office. He went home, ate his dinner, went into his study, and worked until he went to bed. So far as I know, he spent his weekends the same way. I suppose he took vacations. I don't remember any.

Outside Interests

His hobbies were golf and the stock market. He was no good at either one. On the golf course he spent half the time looking for his ball. He consistently lost in the stock market but was wise enough to turn over some of his investments to Mary.

After he left Chicago in the 1960s, he moved several times. Each time, Mary bought the house. Ray said that he never saw any of them until he moved in.

Value System

As mentioned above, Ray looked at life and relationships through the eyes of a Southern politician. In economics, he believed in free enterprise, but at the same time he had a pragmatic view of government as an essential and potentially constructive part of society. He was an early supporter and potentially constructive part of the political process. He was an early supporter of Medicare. I think that was because he saw that hospitals were not going to survive without it.

He was uncomfortable with concepts of values. I remember arguing during our after-work sessions that many administrative decisions were mainly value judgments, trying to make the point that managers had an important role in that area. He never accepted that. He recognized that there were broad social values which formed institutions and served as constraints on their behavior. Within those, he saw management as the process of establishing and achieving goals.

We also argued about what was then the American College of Hospital Administrators. As a young iconoclast, I couldn't see what its purpose was. I thought it presumptuous for hospital administrators to pretend they were professionals, like doctors and lawyers, and College status didn't seem to affect your salary or help you get a job.

The argument never came to a conclusion. I can see now that for Ray, the considerations were political and therefore instinctive and self-evident, not something to theorize about. I was too obtuse to understand that, and he didn't know how to explain it.

Of course, he believed in abstract values like honesty, fairness, and justice, but mostly he believed in the middle-class virtues of order, ambition, discipline, and hard work. He sought power, respected the people who had it or could grant it, and didn't concern himself much with anybody else.

That is not to say that he was hard-hearted. But he did believe that sentimentality was a sign of weakness and was therefore careful never to display any. I always suspected that deep inside he was a sentimental person, but he clearly had that part of him tightly locked up somewhere.

University Politics

In considering how Ray made out in the rugged world of university politics, several facts should be kept in mind: At the time Ray was Superintendent of the University of Chicago Clinics, he was responsible to the Dean of the medical school. The Dean was strong and highly respected, and the faculty of medicine was politically stable. The hospital was financially self-supporting and did not have to compete within the University for money.

When Ray was made Director of the Graduate Program in Hospital Administration at the University of Chicago, the Graduate School of Business was weak and paid little attention to the program. This gradually changed as the university undertook to strengthen the G.S.B. The M.B.A. was a two-year program, and when the faculty complained about counting the hospital administration residency as a second academic year, it was abolished, and hospital administration students spent two years on campus like all other G.S.B. students.

The point is that at Chicago, Ray was not very much involved in university politics. There was not much in the hospital for academic people in the university to meddle in, and whoever might try had to deal with a strong Dean and medical faculty from which Ray enjoyed firm support.

The Graduate School of Business saw the Program in Hospital Administration as a source of tuition revenue. It put no money in the Program and left things at that. Serious involvement from the G.S.B. faculty came long after Ray had left.

Boston

Ray's job at Boston was to develop some kind of formal relationship among three proud, fiercely independent, Harvard-affiliated teaching hospitals and consolidate them into new facilities. Ray was recruited to this post by Bob Ebert, Dean of the Harvard Medical School, who had been on the Medical School faculty at the University of Chicago during Ray's time there.

When Ray went to Boston, he was universally recognized everywhere else as the number one national figure in hospital administration. Unfortunately, that did not count for very much in the Boston Brahmin culture of which Harvard is the center. He applied for membership in The Country Club, and they turned him down.

The organization Ray went to head was called The Affiliated Hospitals Center (AHC). It had originally been formed by (1) the Peter Bent Brigham Hospital; (2) the Boston Hospital for Women (itself a result of a merger between the Boston Lying-In and the Free Hospital for Women, the latter a small gynecology hospital in Brookline; (3) the Robert Breck Brigham Hospital (specializing in Arthritis, i.e., Orthopedics and Immunology; (4) Children's Hospital; and (5) Massachusetts Eye and Ear Infirmary.

Each of these hospitals was in need of new facilities, and collaborative efforts were coming into vogue. Except for Children's (and possibly the Peter Bent Brigham), each was too small and specialized to have a future by itself. The Massachusetts Eye and Ear Infirmary was and is adjacent to Massachusetts General.

If the new organization had five members, there were at least ten different views of its purpose. Bob Glaser, formerly Dean at Colorado, was recruited to be the first head. He got an architect, Bertrand Goldberg, hired to design something (nobody knew exactly what), did a lot of studies, made a lot of proposals, held a lot of meetings, gave up, and left to head another medical school.

As time went on, it seemed that the main interest of Children's and Eye and Ear was related to their respective specialties. As the direction of the project clarified, they dropped out, leaving the other three.

A hiatus followed Glaser's departure during which the three remaining hospitals took over and Ray was recruited from Duke.

After the 1967 Duke Symposium ended one noon, Ray invited me to his office. My plane did not leave until later that afternoon. His move to Boston had been announced, and so we visited about that and other things between phone calls. When it came time for me to go, I stood up and said that I had been at Kentucky nearly ten years, and if he came to need a deputy in

Boston, he might give me a call. He said sit down. In the next ten minutes it was decided that if he could arrange the financing, I would join him in Boston. I went in March of 1968.

By the time I got there, he, Bob Ebert, and the AHC President, the late F. Stanton Deland, had persuaded Tom Cabot, patriarch of the Cabot family and a Harvard graduate and loyal supporter, to head a $25 million fund drive. Thanks to Tom's energy and persistence, and with only a very general idea about what the money would be used for, the fund drive succeeded. It was a key strategic move, because it meant that nobody wanted to be responsible for the failure of the project and for giving the money back.

There ensued a lot of talk and architectural planning. The three hospitals wanted to join in new facilities but were adamant on keeping their individual identities, corporate and otherwise. Goldberg drew all kinds of plans with three towers, but of course there was no agreement as to what would happen in the base structure. Weeks of lawyers' time were spent trying to figure out who would own it and how.

It may be interesting to note that the insistence on independence and identity came mostly from the trustees. Due to the academic structure of the medical school, only two medical staff departmental headships overlapped, and one of them was clearly senior to the other. The administrators were generally supportive.

In Boston, institutional affiliation is an important element of the social structure. Certain people, often certain families, have long identification as donors, corporate members, and trustees of particular hospitals, schools, and museums. People did not want to give that up.

The only vacant land available for the project itself was the Peter Bent Brigham parking lot, and it would not accommodate the kind of sprawling, three-headed structure being visualized. So it was decided that Harvard (nobody else had enough money) would buy up the old, wooden, three-decker houses located across the street from the hospital, and that the new hospital would be built on that land, plus the big vacant property that Harvard owned behind the three-deckers.

Several properties were purchased and a few torn down when Harvard was hit by the student uprisings of that era. Harvard College is in Cambridge, but the medical school is in Boston, next to the Peter Bent Brigham and Children's. The medical students needed a cause and, with the aid of some crusading reporters from the *Boston Globe*, adopted this project of community destruction and the eviction of workers from their homes.

Harvard and the Boston families who patronize it have been around for a long time. They have seen these things come and go. They react with a combination of private verbal indignation and public patience. They never lose their cool. It wouldn't be proper. Ray came from North Carolina, where people knew their place, by way of Chicago, where Mayor Daly knew how to deal with disruptive people, and this tongue-clucking approach was far outside whatever range of tolerance Ray had for such things. On top of his other frustrations, it was just too much.

Ray started to have some phone conversations with his office door shut, and I suspected what was up. He then began to tell me of some things he was considering, so I knew for sure.

Being of another generation and background, I saw things somewhat differently. I confess to some sympathy for the neighborhood people. The institutions, in my mind, were living by the rules of another era. I had to come to believe strongly in these hospitals, and to be convinced that adjustment to the current environment was essential for their continued success. If the properties had been essential for their survival, that would have been one thing. But as it was, they were still arguing with each other about identity, had not settled on any feasible scheme, and just went ahead and started tearing down the houses anyway.

As it has turned out, the three-deckers are still standing, and a subsidized housing project has been built on the big vacant property. The new hospital ended up on the Peter Bent Brigham parking lot, plus a small piece of adjacent land bought from Children's.

Ironically, it was Ray who taught me (and many others) that an institution is the product of its environment. Any reading of Harvard culture and Massachusetts politics at the time would have made it clear that egalitarianism was popular, at least for the time being, and that if you wanted to make the project go, you had to do it in the context of the situation in which it existed. Ray opted not to do that.

One day a year or two later, I went to seek advice from one of the corporation members who operated a successful dairy products plant in the middle of Somerville, a poor area. At the end of the conversation he said "Dick, you go back over there, put your pride in your pocket, get ready to eat some gravel, and deal with those folks. You'll find out it's not so bad." I did what he said and found that he was right.

Under different circumstances, Ray most likely would have done it, too. While the culture gap would have been big for him, he had the ambition, the intellect, and the instincts needed to overcome it.

But by that stage of his life, he didn't have to. It would have been agony for him, and success would have added only a little to his already illustrious career. Harvard-affiliated hospitals had never joined the world of nonphysician hospital administrators that Ray represented, and it is to his credit that he had the good sense to see that.

My interests were different, however, and I decided that if Ray left and they offered me the job, I would take it. During the 1969 AHA convention in Chicago, I got a call from The Affiliated Hospitals Center Board President, who told me Ray had resigned and offered me the job, which I accepted.

Ray seemed surprised but took it with good grace and wished me the best of luck. As to how it got done, I would say that whereas my predecessors had tried to succeed through strength of personality and leadership, I saw the development as inevitable. But only if attention could be kept on the reality that these outstanding institutions had started to decline and that this process would accelerate unless the new project went forward. In essence, I decided to build on Ray's teaching and let the environment take its course while trying to keep the process orderly, not doing anything dumb, avoiding diversions irrelevant to the goal, and not becoming an issue myself.

The final catalyst was the Massachusetts Certificate of Need law. As soon as it was adopted, we applied but, of course, being three hospitals, had to submit three applications. It was hard to make the explanations much clearer than the concept itself. There was a big dinner with the Commissioner of Health who, in a gentle way, made it clear that we might get approval for one new hospital, but hardly for something that was partly one and partly three without being able to tell exactly which part was which. The dreaded word merger was not mentioned, but the implication was clear enough.

The moment of decision occurred shortly thereafter. At the end of a long board meeting, with everyone anxious to go home, I said that unless there was objection, I planned to prepare a single application for a hospital to be owned and operated by AHC. Following a pregnant silence, the Chairman asked if there was any other business and, there being none, adjourned the meeting.

Of course, the entire process included innumerable board meetings, medical committee meetings, community meetings, public hearings, newspaper articles, bylaw drafting sessions, merger votes and all the rest, but as long as we kept the focus on the goal, nobody had the will to kill the project. The Brigham and Women's Hospital (the new name for AHC) is now operating very successfully in modern facilities on Frances Street in Boston.

CHAPTER EIGHT

BACK TO CHICAGO—NORTHWESTERN UNIVERSITY

Robert M. Cunningham, Jr.

The uncertainties Ray Brown encountered when he arrived at Northwestern University were at least as formidable as those he left behind at Harvard. Ray was executive vice-president of the University's medical center, an entity that was difficult to define at the time. The two principal teaching hospitals, Wesley Memorial and Passavant Memorial, were located on opposite corners at the intersection of Superior Street and Fairbanks Court on Chicago's Near North Side. An undistinguished parking garage occupied a third corner, which was seen at the time as the eventual site of a putative women's hospital. Passavant and Wesley had separate traditional boards of trustees, women's boards, administrations and medical staffs—the only variation being that the departments of surgery and anesthesiology had chiefs in common. The remainder of the medical staffs were competitive, not to say antagonistic, toward each other.

The medical center of which Ray was executive vice-president existed on paper and in the minds of a few visionaries in the University administration and a generous benefactor whose initial gift of $10 million to the medical center arrived a month or two before Ray did, but the center in fact remained to be created. The downtown campus of the university consisted of the medical school and hospitals and the university's evening classes and law school. The main campus, undergraduate college, academic departments, and principal focus of interest were all located on the lakefront in Evanston, immediately north of the Chicago city limits.

This is not to say there were no pressures for consolidation or coordination of the medical components, but only to suggest the complexities that had to be resolved—the task, in other words, that confronted Ray Brown when he arrived on the scene. The most urgent of the pressures were in graduate medical education, responding to the growing demand for hospital expansion, rapidly growing health insurance, and the burgeoning demand for training in the multiplying medical specialties. Passavant had already outgrown the original building completed in 1928, a hospital addition east of the original site, and an adjoining doctors' office building to the south. Wesley, which had moved from a South Side location a few years earlier, was spilling over into neighboring structures along Superior Street. The medical center concept also included the Evanston Hospital, a venerable and superior suburban community institution a few blocks from the university campus, Children's Memorial Hospital on Chicago's North Side a mile north of the medical school, the Rehabilitation Institute, recently moved to a medical school campus location, the yet-to-be-built women's hospital, and, in a different sense altogether but still included in the graduate medical education program, the Veterans Administration's Lakeside Hospital, a block south of Passavant.

Following studies by a medical education consultant, the medical center had been incorporated in 1966, with Wesley, Passavant, Evanston, and Children's Memorial hospitals and the Rehabilitation Institute as members and the Veterans Administration hospital as an associate member. The Chicago Maternity Center, a service then located on the West Side and later part of the women's hospital at the medical center site, was also an original member. All members of the hospital staffs were medical school appointments, but the remote sites of Evanston and Children's obviously resulted in a less binding relationship than the ones afforded by the medical center locations. Dr. Richard Young, then dean of the medical school, had served as part-time executive. His appointment followed the recommendation of a management consultant to focus responsibility for leadership and coordination of planning and direction of the planning and development of central and shared services. The consultant also suggested that "the individual selected must be able to bridge the relationships between hospitals and the university and bring them together." It was a goal that nobody would quarrel with, and nobody could define.

Foster McGaw, founder and long-time president of the American Hospital Supply Corporation and a trustee of the university, was the benefactor who had given $10 million shortly before Ray came, and a measure of Ray's success at what turned out to be a monumental task of leadership was the fact that Mr. McGaw gave the medical center another $10 million in 1972. Whatever the consultant may have meant by "bridging the relationships and bringing the hospitals and the university together," Ray Brown had accompanied it to the satisfaction of Mr. McGaw, whose name the medical center now officially bears.

In any case, the first step in bridging and bringing together was the urgent need for support and integration of the graduate medical education programs at the medical center hospitals. As evidence of the need, a medical school publication had indicated that the number of graduate education positions filled as a percentage of positions offered by the hospitals had declined steadily over the preceding 15 years—a clear warning of deteriorating quality. A framework for integration of the hospital and medical school programs had been established in formation of a Clinical Training Committee with representatives of all the hospital departments of ophthalmology, where residents were seen as "university based," with appointees rotated through the several hospitals. The committee had also undertaken to standardize house staff stipends and fringe benefits such as housing, uniforms, meals, laundry, and parking privileges—a major item in crowded city locations. A big step was the payment of stipends by the medical center instead of by the individual hospitals. In 1970, the year Ray Brown came, an Educational, Research, and Medical Care Committee approved a recommendation of the

Clinical Training Committee of a statement of proposed principles for a centerwide postgraduate education program.

The principles provided that all approved postgraduate training programs would be administered by the medical school Office of Graduate Education, with certification of graduates by the University, and that each approved program should have an executive committee consisting of the chief of the relevant service in each participating hospital, and the chairman of the corresponding department in the medical school. The executive committee would be responsible for all matters relating to the selection, assignment, and evaluation of individual appointees, and for the design, content, and quality of the training program. Moreover, the principles stipulated that the designated trainees would henceforth be known as Medical Center Residents and not as Wesley, Passavant, Evanston or Children's Residents. The principles also provided that all payments by hospitals should be made into, and disbursements made from, funds established in the Medical School Department of Postgraduate Education. These principles were signed and made binding agreements by all the participating institutions in late 1970 and early 1971—clearly a major step toward bridging and bringing together.

In a report published in 1978, Dr. James E. Eckenhoff, professor of anesthesia and, later, dean of the medical school and then president of the McGaw Medical Center, and Dr. Jacob Suker, associate dean for graduate medical education and associate professor of medicine, stated that

> much of the success of the integrated housestaff program and of the medical center must be ascribed to Ray Brown, whose patient, wise leadership and coordinating abilities, constantly bringing together and urging decision from center institutions and personnel, launched the medical center successfully through very rocky and turbulent waters.

Ray's method in developing the graduate medical education program and the integrated residencies that resulted, and then in addressing hospitals and creating the Northwestern Memorial Hospital that ultimately evolved, was essentially the same throughout: Get the principals involved in the project to meet and talk, and keep them meeting and talking until they find enough ground for agreement to permit some movement. Then keep them meeting and talking until they can figure out how to put some things together. Then keep them talking until it's done.

"It was interesting to watch Ray at meetings," Dr. Eckenhoff remarked not long ago, reminiscing about the merger that seemed so impossible to many and so inevitable to only a few at the time. "He might sit there for an hour and not say anything, as long as the participants seemed to him to be getting somewhere. And more often than not his contributions came in the form of questions that went to the substantive core of what had to be addressed." The Eckenhoff–Suker report relates the sequence of events:

> In July 1971, discussions began concerning erection of a new building on the fourth corner of the intersection of Superior Street and Fairbanks Court. A Joint Task Force was appointed to plan relative to Chicago campus needs. The Fourth Corner Task Force consisted of faculty, staff members, and administrative officials of the University and hospitals, including the mover, Ray Brown. There were seven administrators and trustees and seven staff and faculty physicians. The Task Force met regularly, the discussions were vigorous, and over the period of a year a list of recommendations for the institutions was evolved. The cast of characters representing the institutions had changed appreciably, and perhaps some of the old inflexibilities had disappeared. Suddenly it became apparent to the participants that the simplest route to realize many of the emerging recommendations was to merge the two hospitals.

After a year of discussions that revealed but didn't begin to resolve the endless details of consolidating not just medical staffs but also nursing staffs and all the technical, administrative, management, business, maintenance, housekeeping, supply, purchasing, and countless other functions and personnel, the key movement finally came from the very top, when the two boards of trustees met separately on the same day in September 1972, and acted to merge and create the Northwestern Memorial Hospital. The Task Force and supporting groups continued to meet and talk as they had done before, but now with the compulsion to find answers, not to keep finding ways to avoid answers. Dr. Eckenhoff has a metaphor for the process: "Going out on a cold, windy day, you button the top button of your overcoat as you go out the door," he says. "Then you discover that it's colder than you thought, maybe raining. So you have to button the rest of the buttons as you go." In the language of their report, he and Dr. Suker put it this way:

> The principle has characterized the *modus operandi* of the McGaw Medical Center. Agree upon the objectives, move ahead as if they have been approved at all levels, and work out the details later. The intent to merge was thus agreed upon and consummated by the Boards of Trustees of the two hospitals months before the bylaws of the new Northwestern Memorial Hospital were written, accepted, and approved.

The trustees got to the top button buttoned, and Ray Brown continued with the task of getting people together to meet and talk—with a powerful new incentive to find the ground on which to agree.

Whether the task was as challenging to Ray as it had been when the ultimate result remained in doubt is now a matter of conjecture. Knowing Ray, one might readily conclude that he became less engaged with less at stake in the results of all the talks. Dr. Eckenhoff suggested as much in a 1985 report as president of the Medical Center,

> In 1973, after the merger that formed Northwestern Memorial Hospital, Brown remarked to John Stagl, then president of Northwestern Memorial, that he believed his work in Chicago was essentially over, that his principal projects were now completed, and that neither the Boards of Directors nor the medical staffs of the hospitals wanted to work toward the common goals of a medical center. He saw nothing but frustration ahead and decided he could not remain as chief executive officer. He discussed this with Harry DeWitt, then president of the Medical Center, and they agreed late in 1973 that within the year there would no longer be need for a full-time executive vice president; a half time individual would suffice. This is unknown to most, but Ray's widow confirms the fact that in February 1974 Ray had made arrangements to leave Chicago, return to Durham, and had made arrangements for an academic appointment at Duke.

He never got there. In the spring of 1974 Ray suffered a severe coronary occlusion. After he left the hospital and was recovering at home, he told a friend that he didn't intend to let his illness change his way of life, and he didn't. Dr. Eckenhoff tells what he meant.

> Ray smoked like a chimney...with a long-time history of heavy smoking. He didn't turn a hair when he had his gall bladder removed several months earlier, or even after his heart attack. He went home with strict orders not to do any work, not to go near his office. No serious reading or writing. Complete rest.
>
> Ray lived across the street from me on Lake Shore Drive. I lived at 1242 and he as at 1212. We parked our cars in the same garage, and of course I knew about the restrictions his doctor had ordered him to observe. And on a Friday evening, I think it was, I pulled into the garage at about 7 o'clock or so, and here was Ray, just getting out of the car, where Mary had parked. Ray had a huge bundle of papers under his arm; he'd been to the office and brought home all this work to do, strictly against the orders he'd been given.
>
> I said, "Ray, what the hell are you doing? You've been told to stay in your apartment and deliberately not to do just the sort of thing you've got there under your arm!" He just laughed about it. "I'm all right. I'm all right. I'm all right," he said, and Mary said, "Give it to him, Jim. He won't listen to me."
>
> I said again, "Ray, you ought not to do this." And they went on upstairs. That was Friday evening. Sunday morning, I think it was, the doctor called and said Ray had died.

That was Ray Brown.

CHAPTER NINE

RAY E. BROWN AND THE AMERICAN HOSPITAL ASSOCIATION

Contributing to AHA

George Bugbee

Ray Brown was superintendent of the University Hospitals and Clinic of the University of Chicago during my tenure at the American Hospital Association, 1943–1954. Of many thousands of members he stands out for qualities that would, and did, endear him to an association executive. Some members of the association paid little attention to the AHA. Others were interested as it might advance a career or, sometimes, save their jobs. Ray, without question, knew how an association might be useful in advancing a career but he was unstinting in his willingness to take on tasks, large and small. He was almost unique in this and, certainly, in the talents he brought to such assignments.

Dr. Bachmeyer, associate dean of biological studies at the University of Chicago, was treasurer of the AHA when I reported for duty in 1943. We were acquainted through the University Hospital Executives' Council of seven midwestern universities.

As treasurer, he served ex officio on the AHA board of twelve trustees. The association was fortunate that this group spanned the spectrum of liberal and conservative attitudes toward government and association affairs.

Dr. Bachmeyer continued as treasurer of the association until his sudden death on May 25, 1953. Because there were only so many offices for members of the association, it was important that assignments be spread throughout the hospital field; with more that 3,000 member hospitals, there were plenty of aspirants for appointments. Because Art was treasurer, Ray did not move to a policymaking position during my early years. However, he was repeatedly called on for help. He had the desirable quality of always accepting assignments, even though they might be time-consuming. He seemed able to do this without damaging his hospital situation. Parenthetically, a number of officers spent so much time on association affairs that they lost their home jobs. Sometimes I thought that that was coming anyway, and association work and time away from the hospital gave their boards of trustees an excuse to act.

Ray was not without some AHA connections and was good enough to accept a number of jobs with low visibility. In 1947, he was on the Committee on Air Sterilization and Air Conditioning. In 1948, he was chairman of the committee to develop a manual on admitting practices and that same year was chairman of a committee on governing boards. Not until 1951 did he have assignments that permitted involvement in the formulation of association policy. That year he was on the Council on Government Relations, an important appointment. Beginning in 1952, he was chairman of the Council on Association Services, which made him a member of the coordinating council of AHA.

During this period, Ray began to write and speak to many groups of hospital and business executives. Often I thought he had formulated his thinking as a faculty member and director of the Graduate Program in Hospital Administration at the University of Chicago. He was unusually good speaking and writing about management behavior. His articles were among the best available from members for publication in *Hospitals*, the journal of AHA.

Prior to taking the position with AHA, I was commissioner–superintendent of Cleveland City Hospital. This was a 1,509-bed hospital and a fascinating administrative assignment. I not only liked the authority but made good use of the opportunity to compare practices with the University Hospital in Ann Arbor. During those five years there were many distractions from day-to-day supervision in the hospital. City purchasing and acquisition of personnel under civil service law were time-consuming, as was dealing with other branches of government in City Hall.

I liked day-to-day operations and came to the conclusion that there were checkpoints that permitted the administrator, when short of time, to see that the hospital was operating satisfactorily. Ray Brown and I discussed this "checkpoint supervision"; he thought it might be possible to develop a manual useful generically in hospital administration. Later, Ray and an associate produced such a checklist or protocol, published by the American College of Hospital Administrators and titled *Hospitals Visualized.*

This was a good first effort, but the checklists were restricted to the less complicated aspects of hospital administration. Work with medical and nursing staff and board of trustees was not included. Years later, when Dr. Edwin Crosby was president of AHA, he hired Richard Johnson, Ray's co-author, under a $750,000 grant from the Ford Foundation to develop a protocol for judging the effectiveness of hospital operations. Eventually, I found that document useful for students in the practicum of the University of Chicago Graduate Program in Hospital Administration. Each student was assigned a hospital. His study and a written report flowed from using the outline to obtain information about operation of his hospital. The students' written and oral reports gave a very good description of each hospital.

This is only one of many developments that Ray's talents made possible. He contributed greatly to the effectiveness of the AHA. He worked with hospital industries in development of better product lines. It amused me once when Ray, not too modestly, said that he was the best-known hospital administrator in the country. What amused me was that he was quite right. He could have said "among the smartest" and I would have agreed with that, too.

Association Services

James E. Hague

Ray Brown's AHA participation sheet (a document that skeletally describes what an AHA member-volunteer did for the lodge) bears out Bugbee's statement that Ray was willing to help out in ways big and small. He helped revise medical record forms but he also chaired a Committee on Hospital Governing Boards, this during a time when the AHA, with Kenneth Williamson leading the staff, was attempting to determine how best to tap the untapped resources to be found among the members of hospital boards.

His appointment as chairman of the Council on Association Services carried with it a seat on the Coordinating Council (later called the General Council), a unique deliberate level created by Bugbee. In the AHA structure, action started at the committee level and then went on to the various councils, Professional Practice, Administrative Practice, Planning, and so forth. At this council level, the committee work, whether it was a policy statement, an operating manual, whatever, would be reviewed. If approved, the recommendation would go up another step to the coordinating council, consisting of the chairmen of the various councils. Meeting in the presence of the Board of Trustees and always the day before the Board met, the council chairmen would bring a variety of viewpoints to bear on each subject. The chairman of the Council on Professional Practice, customarily a physician, might recommend something affecting nursing, but as the Council debated the issue, matters such as cost and who would pay would be tackled for the benefit of the auditing trustees. It was this power role on the Coordinating Council that paved the way for Ray Brown to become president of the AHA.

Howard F. Cook was the first secretary of the Council on Association Services and served while Ray was chairman. Howard writes that to properly describe Ray Brown's service in that position, one needs at least a brief description of the environment in which he, the Council, and the AHA itself were functioning.

> The hospital field of the early fifties was striving mightily to meet the burgeoning demand for hospital care. The hospital administrators of the 1950s were eagerly joining together

to develop and share information on how best to design a modern hospital building; effectively organize and manage the hospital departments; refurbish, modernize and expand hospital facilities that had been in a state of immobility during the depression of the 1930s and the rationed resources of the 1940s; recruit the best possible employees, and provide clinical training for vastly increased numbers of doctors, nurses, technicians, therapists, and others.

In brief, they were trying to bring modern management methods to bear on an institution—the hospital—in which this had never really theretofore been a consideration. The AHA was the mechanism or umbrella under which this effort occurred.

The Council that Ray Brown was chosen to chair covered the area previously handled by three other Councils, Association Development, Education, and Public Relations, including such activities as membership growth, encouragement of regional and state hospital associations, conduct of institutes and working conferences, provision of a national library service, and increasing public understanding and improving public perceptions of the modern hospital. The Council also served as the Committee on Bylaws and as Ray Brown put it, "the conscience of the Association," a function it carried out by "examination of all association programs to assure that they shall be of maximum benefit to the entire membership, by discussing what new programs should be undertaken and what old ones dropped." This was a demanding but central role in Association affairs for Ray, a bright new star in the AHA world at a time of intense activity powered by Bugbee and fueled by massive (for that time) dues increases.

From this point position as Council secretary, Cook was in perhaps the best position to judge Ray as Council Chairman. Cook writes:

> He brought to the chairmanship . . . a formidable array of talents; a healthy impatience to "get on with the job," and an ability to forecast the future combined with the statesmanship required to get there quickly and with a minimum of friction. His AHA future was to be concerned with such matters as hospital finance and the appropriate roles of the

> federal government, Blue Cross, and others in the hospitals of the last part of the 20th century.
>
> He would be involved with such issues as: (1) the newly-established National League for Nursing and its proper organizational and financial relationship to the AHA and its member hospitals; (2) the development of the first official AHA list of hospitals, and a nationally promulgated set of 10 requirements for listing as an acceptable hospital; (3) the conveyance by the American Medical Association of its hospital register to the AHA; consideration of nursing homes for AHA membership and AHA services—all these issues and more benefited from Ray's broad conceptual perception of the paths hospitals would follow in the 1960s and 1970s.

Donald W. Cordes, former AHA Trustee and winner (as was Ray) of its Distinguished Service Award, had this to say about Ray Brown in the same vein as Cook:

> Isn't it interesting that no one has really risen to Ray's place of preeminence? We have had some very good leaders, but no one stands out the way he stood out above his peers. That is testimony to his superior intelligence, but also his political savvy in knowing how to get things done. James Hamilton had an entourage and a loyal alumni group, as Ray did. But I don't think that Hamilton ever quite achieved the height of effectiveness and imprint on our field ascribed to Ray Brown.

My first vivid recollection of Ray Brown as an AHA leader came when as AHA president-elect he went to Washington in 1955 to make a speech to the Maryland–D.C.–Delaware Hospital Association. I was then editor of *Hospitals,* having been appointed the year before by the then-new executive director of AHA, Edwin L. Crosby, M.D., my former boss at Johns Hopkins Hospital, Baltimore. Ray's talk later became the paper, "The Nature of Hospital Cost," which was published in the March 1, 1956, issue of *Hospitals.* It was in that speech that Ray predicted that hospital costs would increase at about 5 percent per year for many years. I talked to him after his appearance, and he said that while a 5 percent perpetual annual increase seemed frightening, he feared that the figure was, if anything, too conservative. His talk was, as was his wont, in writing for the meeting. I told him we wanted to publish it, and he agreed but said he wanted to get some more "talking time" out of it, as well as to work it over. He asked me to edit it and I did. It was one of many Brown papers we were honored to publish. He took editing gamely. I think that "The Nature of Hospital Costs" was the best piece we ever published. Certainly it brought a new perspective to the description of a hospital problem, a new marshalling and analysis of facts.

When Ray took office as AHA president in 1956, he was the first graduate of a program in hospital administration to be AHA president, the latest in the many changes which have occurred among holders of that office since the first president in 1899. The first five were laymen of varying backgrounds, but starting in 1951 the physician tradition took over and dominated the office and the American Hospital Association for several years. Of Ray Brown's five immediate predecessors as president, three were M.D.s. Ray's ascendancy changed that. The last physician administrator to be president was George W. Graham, M.D., in 1969. Almost all the laymen in the years following have been management trained, usually in university programs in hospital administration.

One other change in previous rules of AHA succession. So far as Howard Cook and I know, Ray Brown was the first person to be named president without having served a stint on the board. His successor, Albert W. Snoke, M.D., followed the same route, an expression of the mutually held belief that AHA's strength really lay in its council structure.

There is a saying, or was around AHA corridors, that "There is nothing as past as a past president." I didn't think that was really the case, and it certainly wasn't true with Ray Brown. Under AHA rules, Ray went on to the Committee on Nominations once he'd finished his three years as a president officer, becoming chairman of the committee in 1960. In that position, he had much influence on the AHA future, with a key role in choosing the top leaders.

The 1950s were full of problems of health care of the aged. The AHA was up to its policy ears in wrestling with that issue, trying to come up with a compassionate, realistic policy that avoided the rocks of AMA intransigence and what would be to many of the AHA's basically conservative membership the shoals of national health insurance.

Ray as an officer, educator, and acknowledged leader was deep in these discussions. During his period of influence the AHA came up with the eminently sensible policy that the aged had more serious health problems than others in the population, were poorer than other sections, needed help with their health care, and federal funds would be necessary for the solution. It miffed some on both sides of the argument, but it was far-sighted then and still makes a lot of sense.

When government did do something about the problem in the Medicare legislation in 1965, Ray was in the thick of the fray. Don Cordes writes of Ray Brown's role on the special Medicare committee considering various aspects of the Medicare Act. His group's charge had to do with payment for hospital services. Cordes writes:

> Ray and the rest of the committee were convinced that payment had to be hospital-specific, and therefore we arrived at the conclusion that it needed to be cost-based. How strange it is in 1987 that that is now a much-maligned view! At the time we deliberated in that debate, Ray was very vocal on a differential payment to the community hospital that did no education of nurses, doctors, and others and probably did a minimum of free work. Since indigent care or free services and medical education at least frequently went hand in hand, we on the committee were convinced that the payment for care of Medicare beneficiaries had to be related to the differentials in cost between those two types of institutions. We also recognized that rates charged by hospitals are fickle; that they bespeak the board and management's desire for profit more that they bespeak efficient management.
>
> Ray always saw the community hospital as an essential social institution deserving of protection from taxes, legal restraints, and undue regulation. He had great faith that the boards of trustees and managers of the county's leading hospitals would be cost effective in their operations.

Conceding that the cost basis "turned out to be undesirable," Cordes guesses that if "Ray were alive and active today, he would be applauding the emphasis on market forces, but he would also be arguing for federal financing of indigent care."

Ray Brown once told me, and Howard Cook recalls his saying the same thing to him, that one of his major errors was in not working hard enough and successfully enough for a quick change in AHA's membership policy excluding nursing homes—they weren't admitted to membership for many years. AHA permitted nursing homes to buy publications and services, but that was it. Ray believed that with few exceptions, usually in the church-related groups, nursing homes were not perceived as health care institutions, and therefore, were beyond AHA boundaries.

He thought that business and industry belonged to free enterprise, education largely to government, and health care to voluntary initiative—church groups and community organizations. I recall that he served on a committee to produce a statement on the voluntary hospitals. I was its secretary. At one meeting, Ray said, "You know, the most voluntary of all hospitals is the for-profit." We agreed, but no member of the committee wanted to come out with such an endorsement of the for-profit hospital as the model for the voluntary hospital.

Charles R. Goulet, until recently the executive vice-president of Blue Cross and Blue Shield of Illinois and a former associate of Ray Brown at the University of Chicago, believes that Ray's major contributions flowed from the whole of his activities.

> As far as I am concerned of the many contributions Ray made to the field, three stand out, and I suspect all were related in one way or another to his work with AHA. . . .
>
> The first concerns the negotiation of the Federal Employees Health Benefits Program. The concept of offering each Federal Employee a choice among program offerings I believe was a major contribution that Ray made on behalf of hospitals, working with the Civil Service Commission in the design of the Federal Employees Program. It is interesting that this approach to providing health benefits to federal employees and their dependents has remained essentially intact, though it may be subject to limitation.

> A second contribution Ray made concerned his calling the attention of his colleagues in hospitals to the plight of the elderly in the late 50s and early 60s. Not only did Ray highlight the problems of access and adequate funding for care of the elderly, but he was also one of the first in the health field to point out the possibility of tying the financing of benefits to the Social Security wage tax system....
>
> Thirdly, contributions as an author. It seems to me these led to major change in the direction of discussions concerning hospital costs on the part of hospital people.... There is no doubt in my mind that his thoughtful presentations were the result of discussions that were taking place within the Councils, Committees, and Board of the AHA.

Ray Brown knew how to turn a phrase. I remember him once writing, somewhat sadly, that hospitals were good at the dashes—acute care—and poor at the long distances—long-term care. He himself proved to be good at both.

CHAPTER TEN

INPUT FROM OTHER COLLEAGUES

David M. Kinzer

My own exposure to large numbers of health care managers over many years gives no support to the notion that the high achievers can be cleanly categorized by personality, intellect, behavior or style. What may explain the job security of one may be what gets the next one fired. Besides, the institutional environments in which health care managers must function vary in the extreme, so it is ridiculous to assume that a single model can fit in all situations. Even Ray couldn't do that, for reasons that I will later relate.

In an earlier part of this volume, on "Turn of Mind" (Chapter One), Ray Brown himself writes about the attributes of a successful manager almost as if he believed there could be a standard model. Maybe it helps if the hospital administrator's behavior pattern is generally in line with what Ray suggested, but it certainly doesn't guarantee success. Ray himself was a living example of nonstandardization of the administrative model. In my experience, there has never been anybody like him. I need talk about only one attribute to make my point—his intellect. He had a mind that cut right through to the heart of a question. He forced the people who worked with him to think with him, to conceptualize their problems, avoiding the nitty gritty. Being with him very long could be tiring. It was like being in an intellectual fencing match. Ray felt no compulsion to say just the things that are comfortable to hear, like so many of the health care managers I have known over the years.

My exposure to Ray was limited to the relationship of an elected hospital association officer to paid staff. In 1959 he served as president of the Illinois Hospital Association (IHA) when I was executive vice-president. I was surprised that he took that job, because he had already held the top elective hospital position in the country in 1955–1956, the presidency of the American Hospital Association, and IHA had to be a comedown. To compound the demands made on his time during his term at IHA, he was serving an overlapping term (1959–1960) as president of the American College of Hospital Administrators (now the American College of Healthcare Executives). To my amazement, he was somehow able to give a lot of time to his IHA job. At first I was a little embarrassed to call him about our problems at IHA, but his lines were open to me. If I couldn't get him in his office I was able to get through to him at his home.

Ray did a lot for me. He was a most perceptive critic of some of my earlier writing. And he was an educator for me, too. In the earlier stages of my career, I was somewhat in awe of hospital administrators and the vast complexity of running "voluntary" organizations where no one, especially not the administrators, seemed to be clearly in charge. Talking to Ray one day, I made some comment about the bewildering number of decisions that must be made in this kind of organizational environment. He took me up on this quickly. "The decisions aren't really very hard or very numerous," he said, "if you have a value system that is firmly in place and the people around you know what it is."

I count this as one of the best pieces of professional wisdom I have picked up over the years, and one of the most useful.

If I had a problem with Ray during the late 1950s and early 1960s, it derived from the fact that he so thoroughly dominated his peers. Before and after his stint as president of IHA, I had a lot of trouble finding elected leaders who felt comfortable about thinking for themselves. Their habit was to check Ray for his opinion on the issue before giving me any advice or direction. Only rarely did they fail to follow his lead.

There is a problem like this, too, with many of the people who used to work for him in management. They still express a level of hero worship that makes it difficult for them to talk about him critically or even analytically. Sophie Zimmerman, who was with him longer than anybody else at the University of Chicago, expresses this feeling perfectly. "Personally," she said, "all during my days at the University of Chicago I realized what a privilege it was to work with and for Ray Brown. There was always a challenge during the pioneering days when the health field was relatively new, with so many developments and changes in progress. I can truly say that everything new, good and helpful that I learned and have used in my own career is thanks to his ability to motivate, inspire, provide opportunities and make possibilities possible."

Like me, these people have difficulty separating the education in Ray Brown from his role as a boss. Another one of his lieutenants, Verne Forsman, talks about "the twelve great and enriching years I spent with him as a student, a resident and as assistant administrator at the University of Chicago Clinics."

Though I never had the opportunity to work with Ray as a management subordinate as these two people did, I did over the years get to know most of his key lieutenants, some on a close personal basis. It is their opinions that provide the substance for this summary. University of Chicago people are the heaviest ingredient in this mix, because running that university's hospital and clinics was the last institutional management job Ray ever held. It is often not recognized that what he did after that, at Duke, Harvard, and Northwestern universities, was not management in the literal sense. He directed an educational department at Duke, and at Harvard and Northwestern he had the job of trying to bring together into a tightened management configuration the hospitals affiliated with the medical schools of these two universities, but without ever being given any line authority over these institutions or being directly involved in the patient care functions.

Colleagues' Input

I had written contributions from the following people:

Charles C. Boone, president of the Spartanburg, South Carolina General Hospital. A native North Carolinian and a long time friend of Ray's, he is a 1965 graduate of the Duke University Program in Hospital Administration. He became assistant administrative director of the Duke University Medical Center in 1960 and was closely associated with Ray as one of the instructors in the graduate program in hospital administration at Duke from 1960 to 1966.

Verne W. Forsman, now retired, a 1953 graduate of the University of Chicago hospital administration program. As indicated earlier, he spent twelve years with Ray in various capacities at the university. Later, he became the administrator of hospitals in LaGrange, Illinois, and Temple, Texas.

Charles H. Frenzel, now retired, former director of the Duke University hospital administration program, who doubled as director of the Duke University Medical Center. When he decided he couldn't do justice to both jobs, he was instrumental in persuading Ray in 1964 to leave the University of Chicago to take over the hospital administration program at Duke.

Charles R. Goulet, until his recent retirement, executive vice-president of Blue Cross and Blue Shield of Illinois, in Chicago. Goulet is a 1953 course graduate of the University of Chicago, when Ray directed that program. He succeeded Ray as director of the University of Chicago Hospitals and Clinics when Ray was moved upstairs to become vice-president for administration of the university, in the process inheriting Ray's management staff.

David M. Hatfield, currently director of the Frontier Nursing Service, in Hyden, Kentucky. A 1958 graduate of the University of Chicago program, he worked for Ray at the hospital from January 1955 to March 1961, starting as a medical records coder and finishing as an administrative assistant.

Irvin G. Wilmot, a 1957 graduate of the University of Chicago program, he worked for Ray in a variety of jobs at the University of Chicago Hospitals and Clinics. He left the hospital as an assistant superintendent to become executive vice-president of the New York University Medical Center. Since then he has been chief operating officer of New York's Montefiore Medical

Center and executive vice-president of Blue Cross and Blue Shield of Greater New York. Now working as an independent health care consultant.

Sophie V. Zimmerman, now retired, earned her master's degree at the University of Chicago in 1957. Starting in 1946, she had jobs as personnel director and administrative assistant at the hospitals and clinics, in its Center of Health Administration Studies, and on the faculty of the hospital program up until her retirement in 1971, nearly always in close association with Ray.

I have collected their contributions under headings that I believe are relevant to any judgments readers may wish to make about Ray as a manager. I add a few comments of my own in areas where I had some close-up views of his performance.

Delegation

From Wilmot: "Ray delegated freely while maintaining a remarkable degree of oversight and involvement without either real or perceived interference in the activities of his subordinates. He seemed always to have an awareness of what was going on in the institution. Department heads were given ample rein within their departments, as were the administrative staff members within their areas of responsibility. Both groups were expected to sense those situations the boss should or would like to know about and act accordingly.

"Ray either made or confirmed all the major decisions affecting the organization. As indicated earlier, he engaged in lots of conversation, was open to ideas and criticism, welcomed suggested solutions to problems; but in the end the decision was his. Consensus decision making in the formal sense had *no* role."

From Hatfield: "One time he asked me to solve a summertime problem of flies entering the hospital when the receiving dock doors were open to deliver food to the dietary department. Strings of fly paper were not effective, so I purchased large downthrusting fans hung from the ceilings just outside the doors. After installation, I invited Ray down to the dock area to see just how effective the wind barrier was. The fans were turned on and the doors opened. The flies hit the down draft and were blown to the ground—where they calmly walked through the doors, then flew away into the hospital. I remember Ray just staring at all this, then laughing and clapping me on the back with a 'Nice try, Dave—what else can you come up with, other than stepping on them?'"

Pattern of Maintaining Accountability

According to Wilmot, "Ray did hold his staff firmly accountable for well understood ground rules developed through a relatively informal management process. He was occasionally disappointed, but I don't believe often. He constantly encouraged subordinates to pursue issues and new ideas. For those who did, he was tolerant and forgiving of mistakes made in the pursuit of these ideas and would defend the miscreant against organizational criticism.

"Other accountability programs such as management by objective were not used. In their place was Ray's informal management style with lots of discussion, coaching and philosophizing around specific operational matters or the broader health issues of the day."

Budgetary Control

From Wilmot: "Budget accountability within the operating organization was rigorously enforced. One simply did not exceed approved expenditure levels—not without considerable prior discussion with Ray and some very good reasons. The 'Blue Book' published with monthly and year-to-date figures was one of the best performance reports in the pre-computer era. It contained all the components of both cost and income with comparisons against budget. In addition, standard unit costs were developed and reported. The cost allocation manual was reviewed and updated regularly by Ray personally."

From Kinzer: "Yes, Ray was good at keeping track of the money, but he was also good in another arena where hospital managers' performances are so often measured—seeing to it that there is enough money coming in to finance the hospitals' mission. None of the hospitals Ray was connected with had any trouble in this department. In fact, there were times back in the fifties and sixties when it almost seemed like the hospital would drown in money even though the university never gave it a dime's worth of support. It was all outside grant money and endowments. Getting this wasn't all to Ray's credit, because he was associated with a university that is famous for its achievements in this area. Still, Ray was a very active party in the process. I attribute this to the fact that, by this time, everybody in Washington and in our state capitol, Springfield, who had something to say about grants knew who Ray was and respected his capacity to produce a good result with the money they gave him. This was only one of the by-products of one aspect of his triple-threat attainment, the political one."

From Wilmot: "Ray was not big on corporate nomenclature, considered superintendent an honorable title and never had more than one associate by that title. He believed in shifting management responsibilities among his administrative group from time to time both for reasons of staff development I think and as a generally sound management practice."

From Boone: "He thrived on controversy and discussion and many times provoked discussion by assuming an outlandish position and then damn near convincing you he was right."

From Forsman: "He could always take an opposing point of view to challenge one's ideas and assumptions."

From Zimmerman: "Understanding what management is, and should be, was a basic thread from top to bottom of his organization—from supervisors to their work forces. This made for a feeling of achievement and incentive for continued improvement by nurturing understanding of the overall goals and involvement on all levels."

More from Wilmot: "Ray was easily and readily approachable by members of the clinical staff and his administrative group. He was not 'one of the boys,' however, with respect to the middle and lower echelons of the hospital. Anyone with a legitimate need to see him was thoughtfully and courteously heard. He never had, nor did he attempt to develop, a direct communication network within multiple levels of the organization."

From Kinzer: "Just as the world is divided between the people who like Los Angeles and the people who like San Francisco, so the world of hospital CEOs is divided between the ones who introduce you to their employees and those who walk right by them without even saying hello. I'll never forget Ray's behavior one time when he toured me through his hospital. I got introduced all around and he took the time to talk to even those whose names he couldn't remember. He was the boss, all right, but he didn't lord it over his people."

Patience With Poor Performers

From Wilmot: "He had the patience of Job. He truly believed that there is good in every person and that, given time, that good will be identified and put to use. At times I think Ray felt that he shared some of the blame for performance shortcomings of others. . . almost as if he slipped someplace in the development or oversight process. People did get multiple chances and, as often as not, improvement did come or an alternative to discharge was developed. He fired very few."

From Hatfield: "He was fair but firm. He would give a poor performer time to improve but if displeased he could give that steady stare, clench his jaw, and the person before him would be in for a tongue lashing and, if warranted, his walking papers."

Communication

From Zimmerman, quoting Ray: "Communication is everyone's responsibility. A systematic and well organized approach is necessary."

From Wilmot, on written communication: "Written memoranda were used with rare exceptions *only* to record understandings reached by other means and for general institutional announcements. He was ever diligent at creating and maintaining a written record of all substantive discussions, agreements and decisions. The letter or memo of confirmation with appropriate copies were integral to the management system . . . Those who knew Ray knew the prolific correspondent, both business and personal, he was. We on his administrative staff had access to the 'reading file,' a continuing accumulation of tissue copies of his correspondences with access time limited to two days, after which the material went to file. Because of Ray's extensive involvement in many segments of the external work, the file was an enormously valuable compendium of interesting and important information as well as insights into the continuing strategies of many activities underway in the health field and elsewhere."

Again from Wilmot, on oral communication: "There were few 'regular' meetings. A weekly session of the senior administrative staff was held each Friday, unless Ray was out of town (not as often as you might imagine). Bi-weekly meetings of the chairmen and deans were regular, with Ray setting the agenda and writing the minutes personally. That was about it for scheduled meetings. Ray did lots of one-on-one and lots of *ad hoc* group discussion. More often than not, an assistant, if he happened to be around, was included in the discussion whether it was germane to his formal responsibilities or not. Lunch in the Doctor's dining room was seldom missed, either by chairmen or those on the administrative staff with a standing invitation from Ray to attend."

From Wilmot: "Probably the best example of Ray's tolerance, patience, loyalty and Christian good will was in securing jobs for students of the graduate program. Several of them, who shall remain nameless, managed to get fired not once or twice, but in rapid serial fashion. Ray continued to work for 'appropriate placement' for them and, for the most part, succeeded in finding a job the individual could handle. Most of us lesser men would not do the same. It might be argued that for the good of the individual and the health field such an approach was overkill. That, however, was not for the times or the man."

From Boone: "Of all the people that I know of who had heavy demands on their time, the one with the most was Ray. . . . One day, about twelve minutes before class time I went up to his office to pick up a book. As I was standing there, getting the book out, this young lad walked in . . . . He said he was on his way from Florida to New York, and someone had told him that if he was interested in hospital administration he ought to stop by and talk to Dr. Brown . . . . Well, as you might imagine, you could see the wheels turning in Linda's (Ray's secretary) head for she was preparing to give the usual excuses about why it would be impossible to see him at this time, since Dr. Brown was getting ready to go to class. Then Ray stepped out of his office. He had left the door open a crack and had heard the conversation. Ray stepped out and introduced himself.

For the next twelve minutes he talked with this young lad. You could hear the eager questions . . . and the responses that were given, totally unhurried. Ray didn't seem to be in any hurry."

From Goulet: "Ray was a workaholic. I can never recall a weekend when I was in the hospital that I did not run into Ray on Saturday afternoon, either walking around the campus to visit some building or department or on his way home. He spent many evenings working at home not only on affairs relating to his job, but also in writing, or on association work or helping others with special tasks."

From Wilmot: "Workaholic? Yes! Ray worked long hours . . . usually to 6 or 6:30 as regular fare with a briefcase for after dinner. Saturday was a 'regular' work day with an understanding that it was okay to leave around two or three. Saturday lunch and the hour or two after was frequently the period Ray 'relaxed' and shared his philosophy and thinking with his staff. This was not an organized event, but seemed to evolve with enough frequency that one wanted to stick around just in case. Although Ray was on the road a great deal, he timed his travel for weekends and nights to minimize time away from the hospital."

Medical Staff Relationships

From Wilmot: "Ray spent a lot of time with physicians. More often than not, it was *they* who sought him out. Within the Hyde Park community, where Ray intentionally located, the social contacts were as frequent as those at the hospital. He was very informal in his relationships and was on a first name basis with all. I believe that many of Ray's closest friends were physicians on the staff, a circumstance which never seemed to interfere with the tough negotiations of academic medical center management."

From Hatfield: "He appeared to deal with the medical staff as a business peer, giving respect to their skills and getting theirs for his. Fortunately, or unfortunately, he had a dean of the medical school to deal with when any major medical departmental issue surfaced. These were sometimes very 'testy' meetings for Ray."

From Goulet: "Ray related to the medical staff very well. He was a very logical, thoughtful person who had a grasp of health care issues that permitted him to gain the respect of leaders within the medical staff. I also have the feeling that his counsel was sought by those who did not feel strong enough or capable enough to make decisions easily. That is not to say he was universally well loved by the medical staff, but then neither were all the various departmental chairmen or section chiefs."

Political Orientation

From Boone: "Ray was not known by his contemporaries as a staunch conservative. By the same token, he was not a wild-eyed liberal. You might say that leaves him as a middle-of-the-roader. Not so. He was anything but. His philosophy and beliefs were such that they cannot be categorized. For his approach stemmed more often from his own thinking process rather than from what he heard or what somebody else thought. On the liberal side he felt very strongly about the necessity of making health care available and accessible. But on the conservative side, he felt that everyone has an obligation to provide for his own needs and not to depend on government or anyone else unless it was impossible otherwise . . . I recall his approach which would have mandated national health insurance for virtually everyone, but managed through private insurance with only minimal federal support."

From Goulet: "During the student unrest with the Vietnam War in the sixties, the University and its board were being called upon to take a stand against the war. Ray argued that the University should never take political stands, but should ensure an environment in which all views could be articulated."

From Kinzer: "The stand reported by Goulet in the point above had its counterpart in the politics of hospital associations. With me and other association executives, Ray strongly advised against identifying with any partisan stand on health issues. As a result, we mostly stayed clear of social advocacy in health as distinguished from positions that related the economic impact, on hospitals and the user positions that related the economic impact, on hospitals and the user public, of a given legislative proposal. This led us to try, not always successfully, to obtain bipartisan support for the bills we wanted passed."

As a Practicing Politician

From Wilmot: "In the university setting, and in others as well, Ray was a superb politician. At home he and Dr. Coggeshall had the university administration under total control. I do not recall an instance over the thirteen years I was with Ray where the university even made a murmur. In fairness, they never had cause. I have commented on the medical staff and Ray's attention to that group. All of us remember the skill with which he, Frank Groner, and Tol Terrell arranged the 'musical chairs' of the AHA and ACHA presidencies for their respective occupancies in serial fashion."

From Goulet: "In university politics he made out very well, with the medical environment, the School of Business, and the administration of the University. The main reason for his success was his logical thought process in dealing with issues. Ray understood issues, I think, before others recognized them, and was able to garner data and facts, and to reach conclusions, and finally to articulate those conclusions in a way that impressed his peers, and thus he gained their respect."

From Hatfield: "I think he did extremely well in university politics. He knew the 'system' and how to work it to advantage. He also knew the players and when to be on the offense or the defense. He was more than a survivor of university politics, he was an enabler within them, a skillful manipulator (in the most positive sense) of resources, whether persons or finances."

From Kinzer: "Amplifying Goulet's main point, I think Ray's political success *vis à vis* his peers in the hospital world relates to the fact that he was such a pragmatic kind of operator. Which is to say that he didn't try to sell his positions on the basis of what he might have thought was right (though, as I have already said, he operated from a strong set of values) but on the basis of what he was sure would work. Then he would proceed to overwhelm any potential opposition with his amazing command of the facts surrounding the issue in question. His peers, who so often must live or die by the sword of pragmatism, were usually overwhelmed. The other explanation for his political success was that there wasn't anyone else around who seemed to be able to give the time or the intellectual energy to the issue in question that he was somehow able to give."

Personal Life

From Kinzer: "It is axiomatic that the workaholics of our world, the 70- and 80-hour-a-weekers, often become obsolete before they retire and too often become burnouts with serious health problems. While it is true that Ray died too young and didn't take care of himself very well after he knew he had a heart problem, it cannot be said that he wasn't able to have fun or have interests that had nothing to do with his career. I for one can vouch for the fact that he was always fun to be with and that he could talk amusingly and knowledgeably about almost any subject under the sun."

From Hatfield: "He did have interests—his family, the stock market (only certain stocks), his big green Packard and an occasional poker game."

From Forsman: "A great administrator but a rotten poker player . . . his wife Mary had him beat."

From Frenzel: "Ray seldom played golf, but on the few occasions when I coerced him onto the links his game was a mirror of his brilliant, complex individual. He swung lustily on every shot. He tried to figure why it went astray and then swung again, equally lustily but with a little different arc. When the game was over, he had a high score, he was tired but not exhausted, and he was ready to do better the next time. Somehow you got the feeling the game had not gotten to Ray Brown but that *he* had gotten everything *he* wanted out of the experience."

From Zimmerman: "He enjoyed life. He loved to watch the North Carolina basketball games on TV. . . . Played cards with close friends and colleagues like Andy Pattullo and George Bugbee. It gave him relaxation. When the students of the graduate program in hospital administration had their fall picnic on the lake shore point, he played touch football as hard as they did, and he had the same energy and enthusiasm to join in and play baseball with them in the spring outings."

Publications by Ray E. Brown

1941

"Hospital Facilities for Negro Patients" *Hospital Management* (October)

1942

"Sources of Hospital Income" *Modern Hospital* (September)

1943

"Developing Authority" *Modern Hospital* (May)
"Maintaining Authority" *Modern Hospital* (June)

1944

"Quantity Determination in Purchasing" *Southern Hospitals* (May)

1945

"The Chaplain is Ready to Serve" *Modern Hospital* (March)
"Professional Fund Raising" *Hospitals* (November)
"Factors That Govern Fund Raising" *Hospitals* (December)

1946

"The Hourly Wage Rate in the Hospital" *Hospital Bulletin* (May)

1947

"Use of Paying Patients in Research and Teaching" *Hospitals* (March)
"Hospital Obligations to the Administrative Intern" *Hospitals* (October)

"Facts on Fund Raising" *Trustee* (November)

1948

"Organization of the Hospital Medical Records Department" *Hospital Management* (June)

"Financing Hospital Construction" *Southern Hospitals* (July)

"Silent Music in the Operating Room" *Modern Hospitals* (April)

1949

"Relationship between Administrator and Engineer" *Hospital Management* (June)

"The Value of Medical Social Work" *Hospital Bulletin* (September)

"Hospital Tensions in Board-Administrator Relationship" *Modern Hospital* (November)

"Eliminating Trustee-Administrator Tensions" *Trustee* (November)

1950

"The Technical Aspects of a Hospital's Departments" *Hospitals* (February)

"The Hospital Bed Comes Down to Earth" *Modern Hospital* (January)

"Double Corridor Plan of Construction" *Modern Hospital* (October)

1951

"El Voluntario de Hospital" *El Hospital* (May)

"Organization and Administration of Clinics" *Hospital Management* (July)

"Clinics" *Encyclopedia* (1950 Revision)

"Payment for Care of the Indigent" *Hospitals* (February)

"Measuring the Pediatric Bed Situation" *Hospitals* (November)

"Pediatric Bed Needs Must Be Planned" *Trustee* (December)

1952

Factors Affecting the Optimum Size for a Hospital (With R. L. Johnson) (Chicago: University of Chicago)

"Music in O. R. Robs Surgery of Terror" (With Joel Williard) *Hospital Management* (December)

1953

"Hospitalization for the Aging" *Modern Hospital* (December)

"Nursing School Accreditation" *Hospitals* (October)

1954

"Staffing at the Administrative Level" *Hospital Management* (February)

"Methods Improvements is Management's Job" *Modern Hospital* (August)

1955

"The Place of the Hospital Association" *Hospital Management* (February)

"The Responsibilities of Membership" *Hospitals* (January)

"Importance of Small Hospitals to the Nation" *Hospitals* (July)

1956

"Factors in Hospital Costs" *Trustee* (April)

"The Nature of Hospital Costs" *Hospitals* (April)

"The Public's Rights to the Facts" *Trustee* (May)

"Causes of the Administrative Failure" *Modern Hospital* (July)

"The Role of the Accountant" *Modern Hospital* (October)

1957

"Hospital Professional Relations" *Hospitals* (January)

"The Hospital and the Physician" *Trustee* (January)

Hospitals Visualized (With R. L. Johnson) (Chicago: American College of Hospital Administration, 1961)

"Value of the Intern Matching Plan" *Hospitals* (May)

1958

"Forces Affecting the Community's Hospital Bill" *Hospitals* (October)

Selection of Students for Graduate Education in Hospital Administration (with V. L. Forsman) (Chicago: University of Chicago)

Graduate Education for Hospital Administration (Editor) (Chicago: University of Chicago)

"The Past and Future in Education for Hospital Administration" *Graduate Education for Hospital Administration* (Chicago: University of Chicago)

"Evaluating the Hospital Volunteer Program" *Hospital Management* (October)

"The Total Hospital Bill of the Community" *Trustee* (November)

1959

"Warning Signs of Administrative Failure" *Executive* (January)

"The Administrator and His Reactions" *Advertiser's Digest* (April)

"Responsibilities of the Hospital Administrator" *Journal, American Protestant Hospital Association* (April)
"Give the Public the Facts About Hospital Costs" *Modern Hospital* (May)
"Seven Deadly Sins of the Poor Administrator" *American Business* (July)
"The Art of Administration" *American Business* (August)
"The Nature of Administration" *Modern Hospital* (November)
"Effective Administration Requires Objectives" *American Business* (December)
"Let the Public Control Utilization Through Planning" *Hospitals* (December)
"What's Behind the Administrative Process" *Modern Hospital* (December)

1960
"Effective Administration" *Executive* (January)
"Controlling Hospital Utilization" *Trustee* (March)
"Executives Who Succeed" *American Business* (March)
"Judgment Distinguishes the Administrator" *Modern Hospital* (March)
"Some Forces that Will Affect the Hospital Pharmacy" *Hospital Management* (March)
"How to Keep Good Judgment from Going Bad" *Modern Hospital* (April)
"Planning the Metropolitan Hospital System" *Hospital Forum* (April)
"Good Judgment is Impersonal Judgment" *Modern Hospital* (May)
"Common Administrative Faults" *Office Management* (May)
"Factors Affecting Prepayment Costs" *Proceedings, Institute of Medicine of Chicago* (May 15)
"The Administrator's Best Traits May Be His Worst Enemies" *Modern Hospital* (July)
"Executive Bad Habits" *Management Review* (July)
"Will Success Spoil the Administrator?" *Modern Hospital* (August)
"National Nursing Problems" *Texas Hospitals* (August)

1961
"What's Behind Rising Hospital Costs" *Journal, American Society of Hospital Accountants* (February)
"Blue Cross-Hospital Relationships" *Texas Hospitals* (March)

"The Administrator Must Adapt" *Modern Hospital* (April)
"What Do We Mean by Hospital Costs" *Hospital Forum* (May)
"Medical Economic Realities" *Medical Annals* (June)
"Leading Without Dominating in Administration" *Administrative Management* (July)
"Winning and Losing in Management" *Administrative Management* (August)
"The Hospital as a Community Institution" *Hospital Progress* (August)
"Dynamics of the Hospital Pharmacy" *Journal of Hospital Pharmacy* (August)
"Struggling with the Status Quo in Management" *Administrative Management* (September)
"Panhandler or Problem Handler in Management" *Administrative Management* (October)
"The 'Leader' Concept in Management" *National Public Accountant* (October)
"Failure Can Assure Success in Administration" *Context* (Fall)
"Seven Sins of the Administrator" *Controller* (December)
"Evaluating Hospital Administration" *Hospitals* (October)
"Winner Does Not Always Win in Administration" *Industrial Management* (November)
"The Hospital Is a Many Sided Enterprise" *Trustee* (December)

1963

"Judging the Administrator" *College and University Business* (January)
"Taste of Failure Can Sweeten Success in Administration" *Management Thinking* (January)
"Administrative Slumber" *Advertisers Digest* (February)
"How Executives Implement Decisions" *Commerce* (February)
"Stress Puts Strain on Administrator's Judgment" *College and University Business* (February)
"The Vital Framework of Area-Wide Planning" *Hospitals* (March)
"Success Can Spoil the Administrator" *College and University Business* (April)
"Seeing the Danger Rather Than the Challenge in Administration" *College and University Business* (May)
"How Good Administrators Get That Way" *Nation's Schools* (June)
"The Whys of Hospital Utilization" *Canadian Hospital* (June)

"Change in Administration" *College and University Business* (June)
"The Administrator Can Overexercise His Best Skills" *College and University Business* (July)
"The Impact of Wages on Hospital Costs" *Hospitals* (July)
"Doing as Important as Deciding in Management" *Manager* (August)
"The Administrator Needs to See the People Behind the Problems" *College and University Business* (August)
"Wages and Hospital Costs" *Trustee* (August)
"Administration is No Place for Perfectionists" *College and University Business* (September)
"Medical Care: Its Social and Organizational Aspects" *New England Journal of Medicine* (September)
"The Public's Attitude Toward Hospital Use" *Hospitals* (September)
"Professional Personality Patterns" *American Professional Pharmacist* (October)
"How Executives Implement Decisions" *Industrial Management* (October)

1964

Nursing Education in North Carolina (Raleigh, N.C.: Board of Higher Education)
"Drug Therapy and Hospital Utilization" *Hospital Topics* (January)
"Why Administration Gets Out of Proportion" *College and University Business* (January)
"Pressures Can Unbalance Organization" *College and University Business* (February)
"Responsibility for Rising Hospital Costs" *Medical Economics* (February)
"The Human Side of Hospital Utilization" *Trustee* (February)
"Stress Puts Strain on Judgment" *Nation's Schools* (March)
"Impersonal Judgment" *Nation's Schools* (April)
"Why Administration Gets Out of Proportion" *Modern Hospital* (May)
"Administrators Cannot Count on Mathematical Certainties" *College and University Business* (June)
"Facts Are No Substitute for Judgment" *College and University Business* (June)

"Administrative Pressures" *Modern Hospital* (July)

"How Administrators Dilute Their Authority" *Modern Hospital* (July)

"The Hospital as an Obligated Enterprise" *Hospitals* (July)

"The Hospital and the Public's Interest" *Trustee* (August)

"Administration is No Place for Perfectionists" *The Nation's Schools* (November)

"The Public Hospital" *Trustee* (November)

1965

"Problems of Fragmentation" *Journal, New York Academy of Medicine* (January)

"The General Hospital Has General Responsibility" *Journal, Protestant Hospital Association* (April)

"Too Much Success Spoils the Administrator" *The Nation's Schools* (August)

"The General Hospital's Responsibility" *Hospitals* (June)

"Accuracy Is No Substitute for Good Judgment" *The Nation's Schools* (April)

"Realistic Recommendations on Nursing Education" (with Howard R. Boozer) *Southern Hospitals* (February)

"Nursing Education and the Community Junior College" (with Howard R. Boozer) *Junior College Journal* (June)

1966

Judgment in Administration (New York: McGraw-Hill Book Company)

"Accuracy Is No Substitute for Judgment" *Education Digest* (September)

"Recommendations for Nursing Education" (with Howard R. Boozer) *Journal of Nursing Education* (November)

"Financial Considerations in Medical School–Teaching Hospital Relationships" *Journal of Medical Education* (November)

Medical School–Teaching Hospital Relations (Co-Editor) (Washington, D.C.: Association of American Medical Colleges)

"The Role and Nature of Judgment of Administration *Hospital Administration* (Winter)

"Impact of Medicare on Hospitals" *Journal of Hospital Pharmacy* (April)

"Financing Medical and Hospital Care for the Aged" *Proceedings, Duke University Council on Gerontology*

"Dollars and Sense in Medical School–Teaching Hospital Relationships" *Trustee* (April/May)

"Medicare's Effect on Six Hospital Parameters" *Trustee* (June)

"The Hospital's Role in Medicare" *World Medical News* (June 17)

"Managing by Anger" *International Management* (May)

Multiple Hospital Units Under Single Management (Editor) (Durham, N.C.: Duke University

"To the Public a Hospital is a Hospital" *Medical Care: Social and Organizational Aspects* (Springfield: Charles C. Thomas, Publishers)

"Medicare: How We Got Where We Are" *Modern Hospital* (June)

"The Hospital Redefined" *Hospital Progress* (November)

"Health Institutions of the Future" *The Journal-Lancet* (November)

"The Expanding Role of Hospitals" *Modern Medicine* (November)

1967

"The Changing Hospital" *Journal of Hospital Pharmacy* (April)

"Health Care Facilities" *Public Affairs Press*

"Hospital Costs—How Much Higher?" *Medical Economics* (June 12)

"Third Party Financing" *American Professional Pharmacist* (August)

"Why Hospital Costs Are High" *Hospital Physician* (August)

The Hospital Patient Outside the Hospital (Editor) (Durham, N.C.: Duke University)

"Redefinition of the Hospital" *The Hospital Patient Outside the Hospital* (Durham, N.C.: Duke University)

1968

"Problems of the Planning Process" *Bulletin, New York Academy of Medicine* (February)

"The Community and the American Hospital" *The American Hospital System* (Pensacola, Fl.: Hospital Research and Development Company)

"The U.S. Hospital: An Industry in Transition" *Pharmaceutical Marketing* (February)

"The Hospital Planning Process" *Trustee* (May)

"The Health Care Facilities System" *Costs of Health Care Facilities* (Washington, D.C.: National Academy of Sciences)

"Capital Financing: Dimensions and Dilemmas" *Hospitals* (October)

Capital Financing of Hospitals (Editor) (Durham, N.C.: Duke University)

"Hospital Capital Needs and Sources" *Capital Financing of Hospitals* (Durham, N.C.: Duke University)

Reimbursing the Hospital (Editor) (Durham, N.C.: Duke University)

"Nature of Hospital Planning" *Reimbursing the Hospital* (Durham, N.C.: Duke University)

1969

"The Role of Churches in Health Care" *Journal, American Protestant Hospital Association* (Spring)

Nursing Education in Georgia (Atlanta, Ga.: Georgia Education Improvement Council)

"Meeting Health Care Costs" *Proceedings, National Pharmaceutical Council* (November)

The Changing Composition of the Hospital System (Durham, N.C.: Duke University)

"The Pluralistic Hospital System" *The Changing Composition of the Hospital System* (Durham, N.C.: Duke University)

1970

"Changing Management and Corporate Structure of the Hospital" *Hospitals* (January 1)

"The Evolving Corporate Structure of Hospitals" *Trustee* (January)

The Governance of the Hospital (Editor) (Durham, N.C.: Duke University)

"Strictures and Structures in Hospital Governance" *The Governance of the Hospital* (Durham, N.C.: Duke University, reprinted in *Trustee*, August)

"Forces and Fallacies Affecting the Public Hospital" *The Tax Supported Hospital* (Chicago: International Health Advisory Council)

"The Plight of the Public Hospital" *Hospitals* (July 1)

"Hospital Trusteeship" *Hospitals* (August 16)

1971

"Role of State Government in Financing Health Care" *Blue Cross Supplement* (May)

Economies of Scale in the Health Services Industry (Editor) (Washington, D.C.: Department of Health, Education, and Welfare)

"Implications of the Health Maintenance Organization Concept" *Health Maintenance Organizations* (Chicago: University of Chicago)

Realigning the Health Care Delivery System (Editor) (Durham, N.C.: Duke University)

"The Health Care Delivery System" *Realigning the Health Care Delivery System* (Durham, N.C.: Duke University

"The Hospital Emergency Department" *Trustee* (July)

"New Pressures on Hospital Will Be Social, Not Technical" *Modern Hospital* (August)

"Definitions of Medical Education" *Journal of American Medical Association* (November 22)

1972

"Decision Making as a Process" *Decision Making in the Hospital: The Physician's Role* (Chicago: American Hospital Association)

Regulating the Hospital (Editor) (Durham, N.C.: Duke University)

"The Rationale of Hospital Regulation" *Regulating the Hospital* (Durham, N.C.: Duke University)

"Health Services Management Preparation" *Education for Health Services Administration* (Ann Arbor, Mi.)

"Disciplines Contributing to Hospital Planning" *Hospital Facilities* (Park Ridge, Ill.: American Society of Anesthesiologists)

"Governance of the Hospital" *Hospital Organization and Management* (St. Louis, Mo.: The Catholic Hospital Association)

"Major Issues in Health Insurance" *Social Security Policy for the Seventies* (Ann Arbor, Mi.: University of Michigan Press)

Hospital Franchising (Chicago: International Health Advisory Council)

"Financing Medical Education" *The Future of Medical Education* (Durham, N.C.: Duke University)

"Issues in Health Care Management" *Journal of Hospital Financial Management* (May)

"Health Management Organization Concept" *Practical Radiology* (June)

"Change and Counter Change in Health Care Delivery" *Journal of Michigan Hospitals* (August)

"Training for Health Service Management" *Hospital Administration* (Summer)